Y0-BSM-703

WITHDRAWN

*Proceedings of the Thirty-Fourth
Annual Biology Colloquium*

The Annual Biology Colloquium

YEAR, THEME, AND LEADER

1939. *Recent Advances in Biological Science.* Charles Atwood Kofoid
1940. *Ecology.* Homer LeRoy Shantz
1941. *Growth and Metabolism.* Cornelius Bernardus van Niel
1942. *The Biologist in a World at War.* William Broadbeck Herns
1943. *Contributions of Biological Science to Victory.* August Leroy Strand
1944. *Genetics and the Integration of Biological Sciences.* George Wells Beadle
1945. (Colloquium cancelled)
1946. *Aquatic Biology.* Robert C. Miller
1947. *Biogeography.* Ernst Antevs
1948. *Nutrition.* Robert R. Williams
1949. *Radioisotopes in Biology.* Eugene M. K. Geiling
1950. *Viruses.* W. M. Stanley
1951. *Effects of Atomic Radiation.* Curt Stern
1952. *Conservation.* Stanley A. Gain
1953. *Antibiotics.* Wayne W. Umbreit.
1954. *Cellular Biology.* Daniel Mazia
1955. *Biological Systematics.* Ernst Mayr
1956. *Proteins.* Henry Borsook
1957. *Arctic Biology.* Ira Loren Wiggins
1958. *Photobiology.* F. W. Went
1959. *Marine Biology.* Dixy Lee Ray
1960. *Microbial Genetics.* Aaron Novick
1961. *Physiology of Reproduction.* Frederick L. Hisaw
1962. *Insect Physiology.* Dietrich Bodenstein
1963. *Space Biology.* Allan H. Brown
1964. *Microbiology and Soil Fertility.* O. N. Allen
1965. *Host-Parasite Relationships.* Justus F. Mueller
1966. *Animal Orientation and Navigation.* Arthur Hasler
1967. *Biometerology.* David M. Gates
1968. *Biochemical Coevolution.* Paul R. Erlich
1969. *Biological Ultrastructure: The Origin of Cell Organelles.* John H. Luft
1970. *Ecosystem Structure and Function.* Eugene P. Odum
1971. *The Biology of Behavior.* Bernard W. Agranoff
1972. *The Biology of the Oceanic Pacific.* John A. McGowan
1973. *The Biology of Tumor Viruses.* Joseph W. Beard
1974. *Chromosomes: From Simple to Complex.* Edward Novitski

The Biology of Tumor Viruses

Proceedings of the Thirty-fourth
Annual Biology Colloquium

Edited by
GEORGE S. BEAUDREAU and STANLEY SNYDER

Corvallis:
OREGON STATE UNIVERSITY PRESS

COLORADO COLLEGE LIBRARY
COLORADO SPRINGS,
COLORADO

Library of Congress Cataloging in Publication Data

Biology Colloquium, 34th, Oregon State University, 1973.
    The biology of tumor viruses.

    (Proceedings of the Annual Biology Colloquium; 34th)
    Includes bibliographies.
    1. Oncogenic viruses—Congresses.   I.   Beaudreau, George S., 1925-
II.   Snyder, Stanley.   III.   Oregon. State University, Corvallis.   IV.   Title.
V.   Series: Biology Colloquium, Oregon State University.
Proceedings of the Annual Biology Colloquium; 34th.
QH301.B43   34th [QR372.06]   574′ .082s[576′ .6484]   76-6965
ISBN 0-87071-173-3

© 1976 by the Oregon State University Press

Printed in the United States of America

574
B521a
1973

Contents

Oncogenicity of Avian Tumor Viruses

JOSEPH W. BEARD and DOROTHY BEARD[*]
Department of Surgery
Duke University Medical Center
Durham, North Carolina

THE PURPOSE of this discussion is to consider some essential principles of pathogenesis and oncogenesis of the avian tumor viruses. This subject is of increasing importance for several reasons. In contrast to earlier opinions, there is now no question that the occurrence of tumors in many animal species is the direct result of infection with virus entities (Beard, 1963a; Bryan et al., 1967; Gross, 1970). It is clear, nevertheless, that tumor formation and the morphologic aspects of the neoplasms are by no means related solely to virus influence. Oncogenic filterable agents cause changes in the morphology and growth characteristics of cells in tissue culture, but, in comparison with neoplasms in the intact host (Enders, 1964), cell alterations *in vitro* are insignificant. It is thus evident that the actual tumors are the result of the respective interactions of the virus and the host directed by distinctive determining factors of both. With the present considerable knowledge of the avian virus tumors and their etiologic agents, it is now feasible to note some elements of specific contributions of the interactants to the form of tumor growth.

Intensive studies (Beard, 1963a,b, 1968; Vogel et al., 1969) have shown that neoplasms of the chicken comprise a broad array of growths induced by a large family of etiologic agents closely related in immunological (Eckert, et al., 1964; Sarma, et al., 1964; Tozawa et al., 1970), structural (Beard, 1973), biochemical, and biological (Vogt, 1965) properties. Despite great variations in host

[*] Present address: Life Sciences Research Laboratories, Life Sciences, Inc., St. Petersburg, Florida 33707.

response to these viruses, the agents studied can be arranged in four groups (Fig. 1) which differ significantly in major aspects of oncogenic potentials.

From the earliest studies of oncogenic viruses in chickens, there appeared to be evidence of at least two kinds of agents—sarcoma viruses and leukosis viruses. One caused a variety of solid tumors

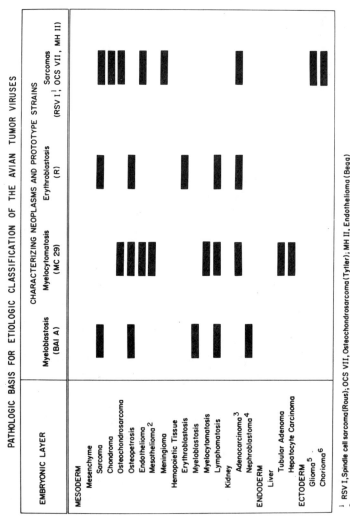

Figure 1. Spectrums of neoplastic growths induced by the four prototype classes or groups of the avian tumor viruses. From Beard, 1973.

(Claude and Murphy, 1933; Rous, 1935), whereas the other, consisting of more numerous individual agents or "strains," produced leukemia (Ellermann, 1923; Olson, 1940; Engelbreth-Holm, 1942) which was often associated with various kinds of solid tumors. At the time, it was common practice to refer to one group as the sarcoma viruses, different strains of which were found to be responsible for fibrosarcomas, chondromas, and other conditions (Rous, 1935), including bone in the very complex osteochondrosarcoma. Infection with the other group of agents (leukosis viruses) was encountered much more frequently in the field (Ellermann, 1923; Olson, 1940; Engelbreth-Holm, 1942; Fredrickson et al., 1964) and was associated with neoplastic conditions of the blood-forming tissues, resulting in (a) neoplastic proliferation of erythroid cells, erythroblastic leukemia; (b) growth of myeloid cells yielding myeloblastic leukemia with high concentrations of primitive myeloblasts in the circulating blood; or (c) a myeloid condition designated as myelocytomatosis (Figs. 1 and 2). Very often, lymphomatosis, comprising a series of solid tumors of lymphoid cells (Olson, 1941) or infiltration of the tissues by lymphoblasts, occurred in birds infected with strains of the leukemia virus group. Those agents or strains affecting blood-forming organs were designated as leukosis viruses, differentiating them from the sarcoma viruses not involving the hematopoietic tissues.

Pathogenic differentiation of avian tumor virus strains

Until relatively recently, interpretations of oncogenesis of leukosis viruses were confused by uncertainties of etiologic specificities. Various strains might produce erythroblastosis, myeloblastosis, myelocytomatosis, or lymphomatosis, singly or in mixtures, including growths of the kidney and other tissues. Points of distinction became evident after intensive studies of a few well-defined strains (Fig. 1). Their characterizing neoplasms provide the basis for classification of the avian tumor viruses (oncornaviruses) into specific categories. Most frequently studied are individuals of the sarcoma virus group, involving a large variety of strains (Morgan and Traub, 1964; Gross, 1970) of the so-called Rous sarcoma virus, some of which induce growths in mammals (Vogel et al., 1969; Gross, 1970). Some of these strains affect cells of ectodermal derivation (Rabotti et al., 1966; Bigner et al., 1969), producing such tumors as astrocytoma, ependymoma, and ganglioglioma. This behavior is not shared by strains of the leukosis virus group.

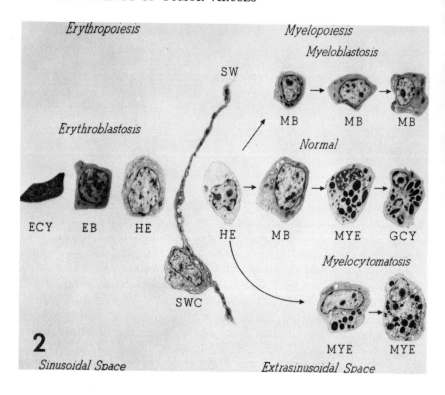

Figure 2. Semidiagrammatic illustration of normal and virus-induced neo-plastic hemopoiesis in the avian bone marrow. The symbol (SW) indicates the sinus wall, and (SWC) indicates the body and nucleus of the cell forming the wall. In normal erythropoiesis in the sinusoidal space, erythroblasts (EB) are derived from the *intrasinusoidal* hemocytoblasts (HE) and mature to erythro-cytes (ECY). The process in erythroblastosis begins in the same way, but, in the fully developed disease, differentiation does not progress beyond the erythro-blast (EB) stage.

Normal myelopoiesis proceeds from the extrasinusoidal hemocytoblast (HE) through the successive myeloblast (MB) and myelocyte (MYE) stages to the mature granulocyte (GCY). In myeloblastosis, the primitive leukemia cell derived from the extrasinusoidal hemocytoblast is the myeloblast (MB), which proliferates without further differentiation. As in myeloblastosis, myelocy-tomatosis arises by infection and proliferation of the extrasinusoidal hemocyto-blast. In contrast to myeloblastosis, however, differentiation of the myelocyte (MYE) bypasses the stage typical of the myeloblast to attain the granulated, though not mature, granulocyte form. The first element derived from the hemo-cytoblast resembles morphologically the myeloblast but does not exhibit the attributes of the myeloblast (Beaudreau et al., 1960b). From Beard et al., 1973.

The leukosis viruses are separable into three groups of prototype strains distinguishable by differences in their pathogenic properties by host response based on the characteristics of the response of hematopoietic tissues, and by the occurrence of other characteristically associated neoplasms (Fig. 1).

The leukemias

The group of leukosis viruses encountered most often under natural conditions (Engelbreth-Holm, 1942; Fredrickson et al., 1964) and exemplified here by the intensively studied strain R (Engelbreth-Holm and Rothe-Meyer, 1935; Beard, 1968) are responsible for erythroblastosis (Figs. 2 and 3). This form of leukosis may be accompanied by a simple type of kidney tumor and by lymphomatosis after long incubation periods (Burmester et al., 1959; Burmester and Purchase, 1969; Fredrickson et al., 1964). Other infrequent conditions are noted in Figure 1. In early studies (Engelbreth-Holm and Rothe-Meyer, 1935; Engelbreth-Holm, 1942) erythroblastosis and myeloid disease were frequently found in the same bird but might occur separately in different individuals of the same group inoculated with the same agent. Passage and selec-

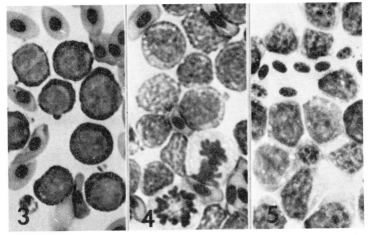

Figure 3.   Typical primitive erythroid cells of erythroblastosis with relatively very large nucleolus, and a thin rim of highly basic cytoplasm. X750.

Figure 4.   Primitive cells of myeloblastosis with granular-staining nucleus, obscure nucleoli, lightly staining cytoplasm, and numerous mitoses. X750.

Figure 5.   Nongranulated myelocytes in circulating blood showing irregular nuclei and cytoplasmic membrane. X750.

tion have resulted in the isolation of an essentially "pure" strain R (Eckert et al., 1956; Burmester et al., 1959; Lucas et al., 1966), which produces erythroblastosis without evidence of myeloid disease.

The characteristics of renal growth associated with erythroblastosis (Fredrickson et al., 1964) differ from those of kidney tumors caused by other classes of leukosis agents. As will be discussed, the occurrence of lymphomatosis in birds inoculated with strains causing erythroblastosis has no characterizing significance. The growth, in all likelihood, is a nonspecific response of lymphoid cells to all classes of leukosis virus infection.

The fundamental basis for clarification of the differentiation of the leukosis viruses resides largely in the results of studies of two virus groups, BAI strain A and MC29 strain. Both strains affect the myeloid tissue, but each induces a different response (Figs. 1, 4-7). The difference between the two types of agents is manifested also by qualitative and quantitative aspects of host response (Fig. 2).

Myeloblastosis, as caused by BAI strain A, is a leukemia (Beard, 1963b) distinguished by concentrations of primitive myeloid cells in the circulation (Fig. 4) which sometimes constitute more than half the total volume of the blood. As a differentiating characteristic, these myeloblasts (Fig. 4) are easily established in tissue cultures (Beaudreau et al., 1960a) (Fig. 6) containing high concentrations of normal chicken serum in a complete medium such as medium 199 with added folic acid, glucose, and appropriate antibiotics. Under suitable conditions, the cells proliferate indefinitely and liberate BAI strain A virus at a constant rate into the culture medium. In the host bird, the myeloblasts arising by infection and proliferation of the extra-sinusoidal hemocytoblasts (Fig. 2) form no tumors *per se*, but permeate all tissues through the medium of the circulating blood.

In contrast, myelocytomatosis (Furth, 1933, 1934; Löliger, 1964), induced by strain MC29 (Ivanov et al., 1964), is representative of another well-defined category of leukosis viruses (Fig. 1). Comparison of the tumor spectrum induced by this agent with that associated with infection with BAI strain A myeloblastosis virus (Fig. 1) shows the relation of the virus entity, *per se*, to the disease process. A major influence of both BAI A and MC29 strains is the induction of neoplasia of the myeloid hematopoietic tissue in the sequence of changes in cell differentiation (Fig. 2). The respective neoplastic responses of both strains on the same cell type are en-

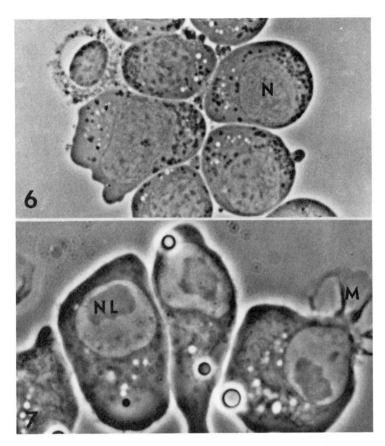

Figure 6.   Phase contrast picture of myeloblasts from circulating blood in tissue culture for 19 days. Cells exhibit internal rigidity with smooth contours of cell membrane and nuclei (N). Nucleoli are not visible. X1500.

Figure 7.   Phase contrast micrograph of myelocytes from circulating blood in tissue culture for 16 days. The cytoplasm exhibits fluidity by formation of large, highly motile external membranes (M). The nucleoli (NL) are very large and prominent, which is a characteristic of most MC29 virus-induced neoplastic cells. X1500. From Langlois et al., 1969.

tirely different. A property of strain MC29 apparently not in agreement with the grouping in Figure 1 has been the induction of erythroblastosis as well as neoplasia of myeloid tissue.

In recent work, however, (Langlois et al., 1971) a component termed MC29 AV was isolated from the standard strain MC29. This component causes erythroid leukemia—erythroblastosis—without evidence of myeloid disease in the chicken. In addition, MC29 AV does not induce foci in chick embryo cell culture monolayers, which is a property (Langlois et al., 1967; Langlois and Beard, 1967) of the whole standard strain. In some birds inoculated with MC29 AV, there were occasional visceral sarcomas and a few cases of lymphomatosis such as those observed in chickens infected with other strains of leukosis viruses. It therefore appears that the standard MC29 strain, as initially isolated (Ivanov et al., 1964), was a mixture of at least two agents, one of which exhibits pathogenic activity typical of the members of the erythroblastosis virus group. Nevertheless, the component that causes myelocyte neoplasms is etiologically specific and, together with other agents inducing myelocytomas, represents a distinct group of avian tumor viruses.

Myelocytomatosis ordinarily is not a notable form of leukemia in the disease caused by agents which are freshly isolated in the field (Mladenov et al., 1967). Signs of the disease in the circulating blood consist of small numbers of primitive cells, commonly designated as myelocytes. Some myelocytes stained with May-Grünwald stain contain a few eosinophilic granules, although the appearance of the cells differs much from that of the myeloblasts of myeloblastosis (Figs. 4-7). Nevertheless, a mild form of leukemia expressed by relatively large numbers of myelocytes (Figure 5) may be produced by virus obtained from repeated serial passages of strain MC29, in birds or in tissue culture, but the concentration of the primitive myeloid cells in the circulating blood is always far less than that occurring in myeloblastosis.

Although myelocytomatosis ordinarily is not marked by large numbers of primitive cells in the circulating blood, there are other manifestations of myeloid cell neoplasia (Figs. 8-10). These include accumulations of masses of myelocytes (Mladenov et al., 1967), varying from minute to large size, which are ordinarily associated with bone. Sites of predilection are the pelvis, skull (Fig. 9), sternum (Fig. 8), and ribs, although other bones may be involved. The growths originate in the bone marrow and expand outward as solid masses of myelocytes with varying numbers of granules colored brilliant red with May-Grünwald-Giesma stain. In the skull, the masses may involve the entire calvarium (Fig. 10) with severe compression of the brain. Myelocytomas occur in relatively low incidence in some lines of chickens and not at all in others. As already mentioned, myeloblasts do not form tumor aggregates.

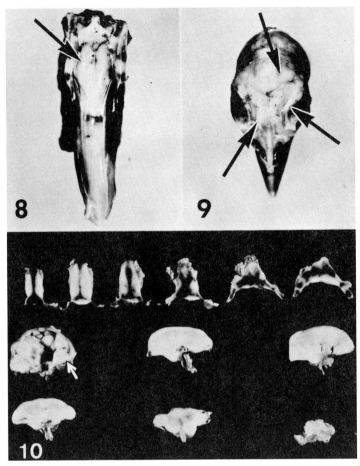

Figure 8.   Extensive myelocytoma (arrow) in sternum of chick diseased with MC29 virus. From Mladenov et al., 1967.

Figure 9.   Massive myelocytomatous involvement of skull (arrow). From Mladenov et al., 1967.

Figure 10.   Upper row of figures illustrates transverse thick slices of myelocytoma of the sternum shown in Figure 8. Lower rows show analogous sections of skull of Figure 9, revealing remaining minute cranial space (arrow). From Mladenov et al., 1967.

BAI strain A myeloblasts and strain MC29 myelocytes differ in their effect on cells in tissue culture. Myeloblasts derived from the circulating blood (Beaudreau et al., 1960a) (Fig. 6) or by treatment of normal bone marrow (Beaudreau et al., 1960b) with BAI strain A virus in culture proliferate enduringly *in vitro*. However, MC29 myelocytes not only do not proliferate (Langlois et al., 1969) but cells harvested from the blood (Fig. 7) or tumor masses survive only a few days in culture under conditions suitable for continuous myeloblast growth. An analogous result is observed on exposure of bone marrow to MC29 virus *in vitro* (Langlois et al., 1969). A few primitive myeloid cells become evident but soon disappear from the cultures. This is a good example of virus specificity in the differential influence of two closely related agents on the same type of responding cell.

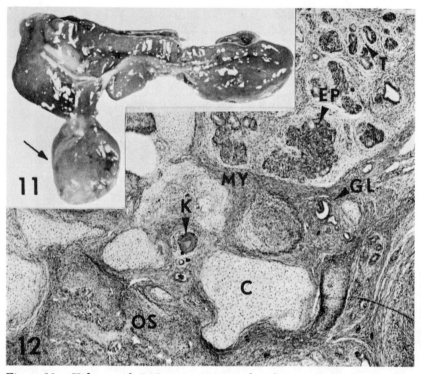

Figure 11.   Kidney with BAI strain A virus-induced tumor (arrow) protruding from the superficial tissue of the organ without invasion. From Ishiguro et al., 1962.

Figure 12.   Survey micrograph of BAI strain A virus-induced nephroblastoma showing much cartilage (C), tubules (T) of undifferentiated epithelium (EP), primitive glomerulus-like epithelial arrangements (GL), mass of keratinized columnar cells (K), osteoid (OS), and mesenchymo-epithelial tissue (MY) from which other structures originated. X5. Courtesy of J. F. Chabot.

Renal tumors

Another distinction between the BAI strain A and strain MC29 viruses in the response of the same host cells to the two agents appears in the differences in renal tumors resulting from infection with the respective agents. Kidney tumor associated with BAI strain A virus infection (Figs. 11-13) is a typical nephroblastoma (Ishiguro et al., 1962; Heine et al., 1962; Chabot, 1970; Beard et al., 1976) with characteristics similar to Wilms' tumor of man. The nephroblastoma arises from nephrogenic cells of embryonal rests located in the cortex adjacent to the renal capsule. It pushes outward (Fig. 11) with relatively little tendency to invade the kidney tissue. The morphology and behavior of cells appear to be in transitional stages of differentiation between primitive mesenchymal nephroblastema (Heine et al., 1962) and epithelium (Fig. 13) destined ultimately to form the normal nephronic structures. Embedded in this matrix of mesenchymo- epithelial tissue are progenitors of all structures constituting

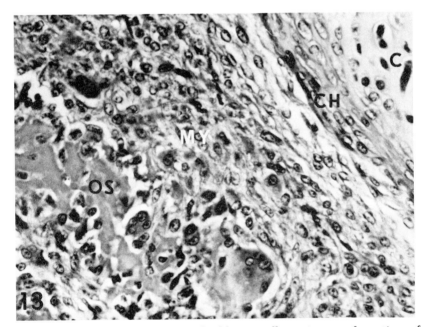

Figure 13. Area of BAI strain A nephroblastoma illustrating transformations of mesenchymo-epithelial cells (MY) to osteoid (OS) in one region and of like cells being transformed to chondrocytes (CH) and cartilage (C) nearby. X300. Courtesy of J. F. Chabot.

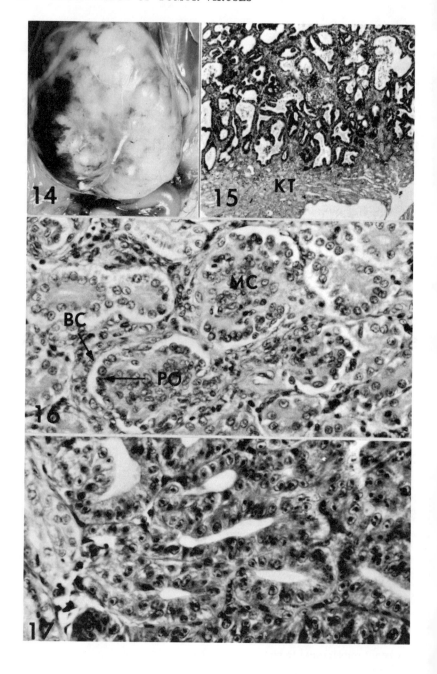

the normal nephron. In some areas, the aberrant glomeruli are difficult to distinguish from normal with the light microscope. Differentiation, however, varies widely and the tumor may contain sheets and masses of epithelial and other cells which have little resemblance to renal tissue (Fig. 12). Metaplasia and anaplasia are common, and occasionally large masses of cartilage and osteoid may be present (Figs. 12 and 13). Sarcomas consisting of spindle cells lying in a dense matrix of collagen develop by systematic transition from epithelial cells. Isolated foci of columnar cells (Fig. 12) may form small masses of keratinized elements.

Renal tumors occurring in birds infected with strain MC29 (Figs. 14-17) differ markedly from nephroblastoma in cell morphology and growth characteristics (Löliger, 1964; Mladenov et al., 1967; Beard et al., 1976). Renal tissues involved by MC29 strain arise from embryonal rests and reach sizes of several inches in length or diameter (Fig. 14) as do, also, the BAI strain A nephroblastoma. However, the propensity for growth into and invasion (Fig. 15) of the kidney tissue by neoplastic cells is different. For the most part, the neoplasms appear as adenocarcinomas (Fig. 17) with a tendency to papillary adenocarcinoma and the formation of poorly differentiated glomeruli (Fig. 16). An outstanding feature is the absence of the basic mesenchymo-epithelial growth regularly constituting the principal tissue of the BAI strain A nephroblastoma, and the presence of primitively differentiated glomerular or tubular cells (Fig. 16). The carcinoma readily invades the cortical and deeper medullary structures of the kidney. Small growths consisting primarily of glomerular tufts or aberrant epithelial strands are very numerous in the superficial regions of the cortex but may extend deeply into the renal tissue. Cartilage formation is rare and occurs only in minute foci. Metaplastic and anaplastic structures common in nephro-

---

Figure 14.   Renal carcinoma induced by strain MC29 showing neoplastic invasion and involvement of total organ.

Figure 15.   MC29 strain-induced renal papillary adenocarcinoma invading kidney tissue (KT). X5.

Figure 16.   Aberrant glomerular tufts with poorly differentiated Bowman capsule epithelium (BC), disorganized and undifferentiated podocytes (PO), and mass cells (MC). X300. Courtesy of J. F. Chabot.

Figure 17.   Adenocarcinoma from growths like those illustrated in Figures 14 and 15. X350.

blastomas are not seen in the strain MC29 growth. Massive cyst formation is a constant feature (Löliger, 1964), and large parts of the growths may be enveloped by huge, thin-walled structures containing a serosanguineous fluid.

Renal tumors are associated in varying frequency with essentially all leukosis virus infections and also have been described (Carr, 1959) as ancillary to growths induced by nonleukosis viruses of the sarcoma class of agents. Such renal neoplasms vary with the virus strain involved but resemble in principle, though not in size or frequency, the MC29 variety of tumor. In some instances the growths are superficial proliferations composed of small cysts. The most significant feature of the renal tumors associated with infection by the chicken tumor viruses thus far described is the unique structure of the nephroblastoma induced by BAI strain A. It is notable that the difference has not been discerned by some authors (Fredrickson et al., 1964; Feldman and Olson, 1965; Purchase and Burmester, 1972).

Mesotheliomas

In foregoing sections the specificity of the related, though distinct, BAI strain A and MC29 virus entities were considered. These two strains may be equally selective in their action on host cells.

Strain MC29 produces a broad spectrum of neoplasms not associated with any other avian tumor virus or any other filterable agent. Among these singular growths is a series of malignant mesotheliomas (Chabot et al., 1970) derived by metaplastic and anaplastic changes of the peritoneal, epicardial, and pericardial serosal cells. After inoculation of MC29 virus into the abdomen, the squamosal cells of these serous membranes, especially those of the mesentery, become rounded and globular (Fig. 18) and may proliferate rapidly to form low or high papillary protrusions. With further growth, many of the papillae coalesce into tumors or expand to form large masses enclosed in mesenteric folds. These may involve the visceral organs, especially the pancreas and duodenum (Fig. 19). Epithelioid cells with large vesicular nuclei and prominent nucleoli usually are compactly arranged (Fig. 20) with thin strands of fibrous tissue stroma. Exposure to virus leaked from the needle during intracardiac injections results in similar growths in the epicardium, pericardium, and frequently the myocardium.

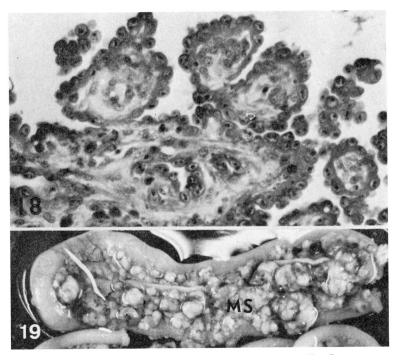

Figure 18.   Papillary transformation and growth of initially flat mesenteric epithelium induced in peritoneum by strain MC29. X350.

Figure 19.   Well-developed masses of separate and confluent mesotheliomas (MS) arising from mesentery about the pancreas and duodenum.

Metaplastic alteration of the epithelial cells to well-developed cartilage (Fig. 20) is found in the mesotheliomas. These changes may occur in the early stages of neoplasia and involve the total growth. The cartilage has not been observed to form bone. Transformation of epithelial cells to chondroblasts and chondrocytes is often so extensive that the mesothelial aspects of the tumors are obscured by the masses of cartilage.

Ovarian tumor (thecoma)

A growth consisting of multiple, stalked, or pedunculated primary tumors (Fig. 21) of the ovary has been observed as a result of infection with an agent derived under special conditions (Veprek et al., 1971) from the BAI strain A virus. Nucleic acid products of the virus extracted in preparations free of the intact agent induced infection of chick embryo cells and liberation of virus into the culture fluid.

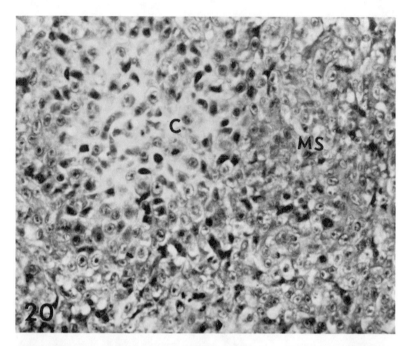

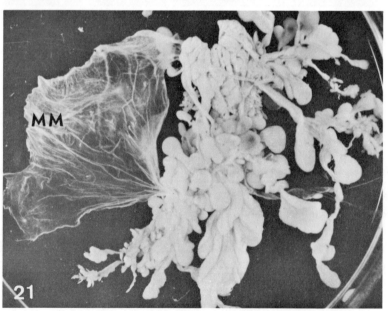

This tissue-culture-derived agent inoculated into day-old chicks produced myeloblastosis with frequently associated nephroblastoma, and, after protracted incubation periods, the ovarian tumors appeared in rather high incidence. Histological examination revealed thecomas, often in association with egg follicles. Such growths have not been observed (Beard, 1968) under other conditions in several thousand chicks inoculated with strains MC29, RPL 12, R, ES4, or with the usual preparations of intact BAI strain A virus.

Hepatoma

Primary malignant growths of the liver are encountered infrequently in the chicken under natural conditions (Feldman and Olson, 1965). Furthermore, potential virus etiology of hepatomas was not recognized until work was undertaken with strain MC29 several years ago. Observations in about 4,000 chicks since 1966 (Heine et al., 1966) have revealed a broad spectrum of hepatic neoplasms (Heine et al., 1966; Beard et al., 1971; Hillman, 1971; Beard et al., 1975). Experimental production of hepatomas can be achieved readily through use of a variety of carcinogenic hydrocarbons (Stewart and Snell, 1957), and growths also can be produced by materials encountered under natural conditions.

These organic carcinogens (Stewart and Snell, 1957) produce a wide variety of neoplasms, derived principally from growth of hepatocytes. Attempts at classification have drawn attention to well-defined trabecular neoplasms, adenocarinomas, and neoplasms resembling malignant hyperplasia of bile duct epithelium. Although some of the growths exhibit evidence of restrained cell differentiation and tissue organization, others show marked anaplasia. Some tumors which are clearly derived from hepatocytes are indistinguishable from primary fibrosarcomas.

Virus-induced primary liver tumors, as illustrated by the gross aspects of the liver of one bird (Fig. 22), simulate in appearance (Hillman, 1971; Beard et al., 1975) the neoplasms produced by chemical carcinogens. Trabecular forms (Fig. 23) and adenocarcinomas

Figure 20. Cells of typical mesothelioma (MS) morphology and structure with area of transformation to cartilage (C). X350.

Figure 21. Tumors of thecoma cells arising in bird inoculated with virus derived by passage in tissue culture initiated with virus-free extracts of BAI strain A virus. A fragment of mesentery floats from growth at left (MM). From Veprek et al., 1971.

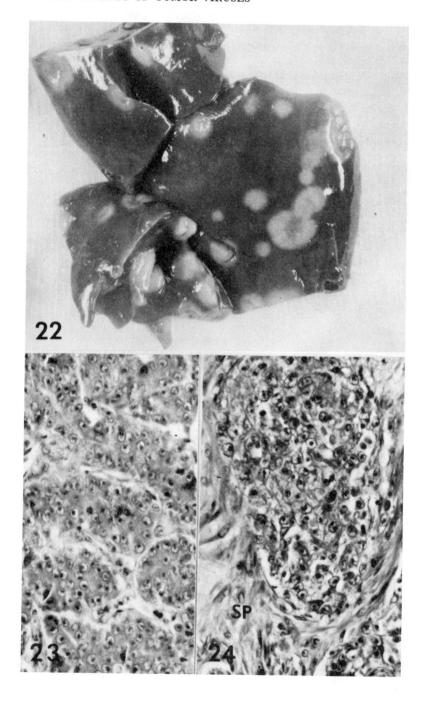

are prominent. In addition to transitions of liver cells to tumors, the growths frequently progressed to highly irregular anaplastic and bizarre neoplasms with complete loss of organization (Figs. 24-26). Further anaplastic degeneration to cartilage (Fig. 27) occurs, but bone formation was not observed. There were also well-developed fibrosarcomas with transitional forms of hepatocytes in the process of transformation from disrupted acinar formations and strands to spindle cell sarcomas embedded in a heavy matrix of collagen.

Pseudobiletubule neoplasms

Growths derived directly from bile tubule cells were not evident. However, epithelial elements resembling duct cells formed growths apparently emanating from transformed hepatocytes. Such cells formed masses or sheets, and frequently mimicked tubules. Under suitable conditions of observation, such as the initial stages of minute growths, the tubule-like cell proliferation arose in the portal septum about the lobule. Trabecular carcinomas originated in the same region, as did many adenocarcinomas. The initial growth origin of adenocarcinomas was frequently indefinite.

Mosaic-type growth

Neoplasms of distinctive types not apparent either under natural conditions or induced by other carcinogens frequently occurred. A prominent condition consisted of hepatocytes transformed into sheets of disrupted individual cells arrayed in whorl arrangements resembling mosaic patterns (Fig. 28). From such transformed hepatocytes, giant multinucleate cells often appeared in the mass of cells of mosaic distribution.

Hemorrhagic carcinoma

Another frequently observed disease was a type of "hemorrhagic carcinoma" derived from adenomatous hepatomas and consisting of cells exhibiting varying degrees of lethal differentiation (Fig. 29) and large cystlike hematomas.

Figure 22. Liver with multiple primary tumors deriving from hepatocytes in bird infected with strain MC29.

Figure 23. Primary hepatic carcinoma with typical trabecular organization of growth. X350.

Figure 24. Portion of adenocarcinoma with advanced tissue disorganization surrounded by relatively thick supporting spindle cell (SP) stroma. X350.

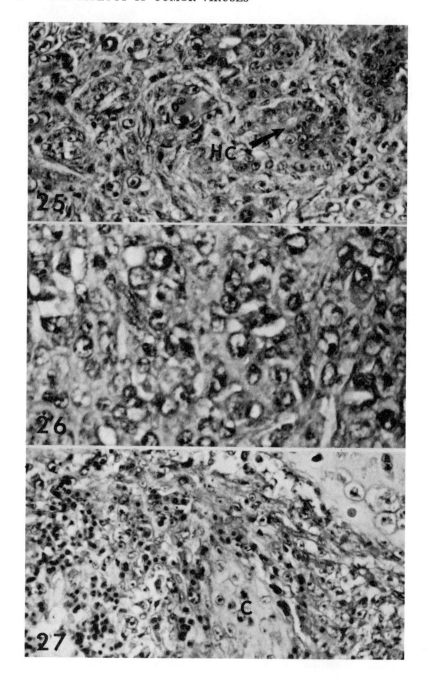

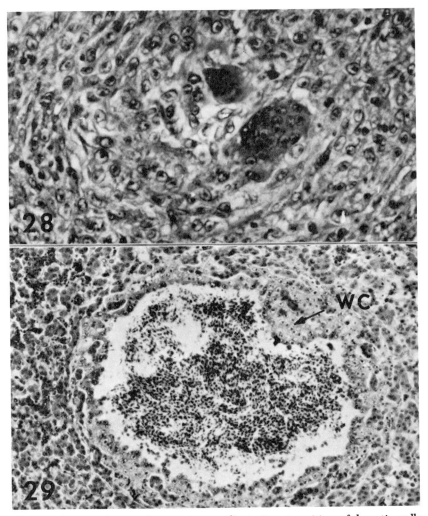

Figure 25.   Anaplastic adenocarcinoma illustrating transition of hepatic cells (HC) in an acinar arrangement to dispersed, disorganized tumor cells. X350.

Figure 26.   Highly anaplastic and disorganized hepatic cell tumor. X914.

Figure 27.   Transition of hepatoma cells of anaplastic growth to chondrocytes and cartilage (C). X350.

Figure 28.   Mosaic tumor with cells free of supporting structure and arranged in whorl conformation with embedded giant cell. X450.

Figure 29.   Hemorrhagic carcinoma with lethal differentiation of wall cells (WC) and formation of cyst containing mixture of red blood cells and desquamated wall cells. X134.

Lymphomatosis

Lymphomatosis is a neoplastic state usually characterized (Olson, 1941; Burmester, 1952; Burmester and Purchase, 1969) by malignant lymphocytes. Growths vary from large tumor masses, chiefly in the viscera and particularly in the liver, to nodular or dispersed infiltrative processes especially prevalent in the liver. Lymphomatosis appears as a relatively late manifestation and is induced by exposure to all leukemia virus strains thus far studied. Since the disease exhibits no distinguishing characteristics relative to the respective activating strains, lymphomatosis is not applicable to virus class differentiation. There is no apparent evidence of the existence of a specific lymphomatosis virus. In this respect, it is notable that strain RPL 12 (Olson, 1941; Burmester, 1952), long regarded as a lymphomatosis virus, is actually a member of the erythroblastosis (Gross et al., 1959) group analogous to that of strain R (Fig. 1). Large mononuclear cells observed in the circulating blood of birds with strain RPL 12 disease (Burmester, 1952) proved to be erythroblasts (Gross et al., 1959; Beard, 1963a) rather than lymphoblasts as earlier implied. Lymphomatosis has not been reported to occur in birds infected with sarcoma viruses.

Summary

Interrelationships between agents of the avian virus tumors have not been clarified despite study of numerous naturally occurring isolates or strains (Engelbreth-Holm, 1942; Fredrickson et al., 1964) derived from birds throughout the world. A principal contributing factor has been the relatively superficial examination of isolates. In consequence, a broad array of neoplastic states of apparently random distribution without definable virus specificity has been recorded. Actually, there are no present criteria for unequivocal identification of a single entity or for distinction of different variations in a given strain.

Some presently well-defined strains were originally mixtures. BAI strain A, for example, originally induced erythroblastosis (Hall, et al., 1941; Johnson, 1941) as well as myeloblastosis, but the erythroid component was eliminated and has not reappeared. Strain MC29 induces not only myelocytomatosis but erythroblastosis. It would appear that strain MC29 consists of two or more agents, and that the plasma of MC29-infected birds contains at least one oncogenic component with properties different from those of any other leukosis virus. The same statement appears to apply to other strains responsible for myelocytomatosis (Furth, 1933, 1934; Löliger, 1964).

Various systems have been suggested (Campbell, 1961; Biggs, 1963; Biggs and Payne, 1967) for classification of the avian tumor viruses. In addition to differences in oncogenesis and in the tissues affected, distinctions in types related to virus particle envelopes have been demonstrated (Ishizaki and Vogt, 1966; Vogt, 1969). Thorough studies have not yet been made to correlate the various strain envelope types or subgroups with pathogenesis. Thus far, however, there has been no definite evidence of a relationship between envelope types and pathogenesis.

Despite the complexities of host-virus interactions of avian tumor viruses, repeated observations with a few strains selected for distinctive differences in behavior have yielded remarkably consistent results in all laboratories working with these strains. As illustrated by examples in this discussion, each strain exhibits elements of pathogenic specificity which are altered only by severe change in the character of host-virus interaction. Behavior of a given strain may be varied, for example, by serial passage in tissue culture or by passage through tissue culture of material extracted from the virus particles (Veprek et al., 1971). Nevertheless, the basic characteristics of pathogenesis and oncogenesis exhibit enduring specificity. For example, strain MC29 regularly induces adenocarcinomas of the kidney but not nephroblastomas. The same strain is responsible for mesotheliomas and hepatomas which are never associated with other strains. Other criteria, such as subgrouping by membrane properties, further characterize and correlate attributes of the strains. As an ultimate goal, final distinctions of grouping of strains and the charting of the finer differences within individual strain classes will probably be dependent on recognition and demonstration of nucleic acid constitution.

Acknowledgments: Preparation of this chapter was aided by Research Grant C-4572 to Duke University from the National Cancer Institute, NIH, USPHS; by Contract Number NIH 71-2132 and Contract Number NO1-CP-33291 within the Virus Cancer Program of the NCI, NIH, USPHS; and by the Dorothy Beard Research Fund.

Literature Cited

Beard, D., J. F. Chabot, A. J. Langlois, E. A. Hillman, and J. W. Beard. 1970. Singularity of oncogenic activity of strain MC29 avian leukosis virus. Archiv für Geschwulstforschung., *35*: 315-325.

Beard, J. W. 1963a. Avian virus growths and their etiologic agents. In *Advances in Cancer Research*, vol. 7. A. Haddow and S. Weinhouse, eds., pp. 1-127. New York: Academic Press.

Beard, J. W. 1963b. Viral tumors of chickens with particular reference to the leukosis complex. Ann. N.Y. Acad. Sci., *108*: 1057-1085.

Beard, J. W. 1968. Introduction to avian leukemia. In *Experimental Leukemia*, M. A. Rich, ed., pp. 205-232. New York: Appleton-Century-Crofts.

Beard, J. W. 1973. Oncornaviruses. I. The avian tumor viruses. In *Ultrastructure of Animal Viruses and Bacteriophages: An Atlas*, A. J. Dalton and F. Haguenau, eds., pp. 261-267. New York: Academic Press.

Beard, J. W., J. F. Chabot, D. Beard, U. Heine, and G. E. Houts. 1976. Renal neoplastic response to leukosis virus strains BAI A (avian myeloblastosis virus) and MC29. Cancer Res., *36*: 339-353.

Beard, J. W., E. A. Hillman, D. Beard, K. Lapis, and U. Heine. 1975. Neoplastic response of the avian liver to host infection with strain MC29 leukosis virus. Cancer Res., *35*: 1603-1627.

Beard, J. W., A. J. Langlois, and D. Beard. 1971. Etiological strain specificities of the avian tumor viruses. In *Unifying Concepts of Leukemia*, R. M. Dutcher and L. Chieco-Bianchi, eds., pp. 31-44. (*Bibl. haemat.* no. 39.) Basel: S. Karger, 1973.

Beaudreau, G. S., C. Becker, R. A. Bonar, A. M. Wallbank, D. Beard, and J. W. Beard. 1960a. Virus of avian myeloblastosis. XIV. Neoplastic response of normal chicken bone marrow treated with the virus in tissue culture. J. Nat. Cancer Inst., *24*: 395-415.

Beaudreau, G. S., T. Stim, A. M. Wallbank, and J. W. Beard. 1960b. Virus of avian myeloblastosis. XVI. Kinetics of cell growth and liberation of virus in cultures of myeloblasts. Nat Cancer Inst. Mono, *4*: 167-187.

Biggs, P. M. 1963. The avian leukosis complex. The Poultry Rev., *3*: 3-12.

Biggs, P. M., and L. N. Payne. 1967. The avian leukosis complex. Vet. Record Suppl., *80*: 5-7.

Bigner, D. D., G. L. Odom, M. S. Mahaley, Jr., and E. D. Day. 1969. Brain tumors induced in dogs by the Schmidt-Ruppin strain of Rous sarcoma virus: Neuropathological and immunological observations. J. Neuropath. and Exper. Neuro., *28*: 648-680.

Bryan, W. R., A. J. Dalton, and F. J. Rauscher. 1967. The viral approach to human leukemia and lymphoma: Its current status. In *Progress in Hematology*, vol. 5, E. B. Brown and C. V. Moore, eds., pp. 137-179. New York: Grune and Stratton.

Burmester, B. R. 1952. Studies on fowl lymphomatosis. Ann. N.Y. Acad. Sci., *54*: 992-1003.

Burmester, B. R., and H. G. Purchase. 1969. Occurrence, transmission and oncogenic spectrum of the avian leukosis viruses. In *Comparative Leukemia Research*, R. M. Dutcher, ed., pp. 83-94. (*Bibl. haemat.* no. 36). Basel: S. Karger, 1970.

Burmester, B. R., W. G. Walter, M. A. Gross, and A. K. Fontes. 1959. The oncogenic spectrum of two "pure" strains of avian leukosis. J. Nat. Cancer Inst., *23:* 277-291.

Campbell, J. G. 1961. A proposed classification of the leukosis complex and fowl paralysis. Brit. Vet. J., *117:* 316-325.

Carr, J. G. 1959. A survey of fowl tumors for induction of kidney carcinomas. Virology, *8:* 269-270.

Chabot, J. F. 1970. Neoplastic process in the kidneys of chickens in response to avian tumor viruses. Ph.D. dissertation, Duke University, Durham.

Chabot, J. F., D. Beard, A. J. Langlois, and J. W. Beard. 1970. Mesotheliomas of peritoneum, epicardium and pericardium induced by strain MC29 avian leukosis virus. Cancer Res., *30:* 1287-1308.

Claude, A., and J. B. Murphy. 1933. Transmissible tumors of the fowl. Phys. Rev., *13:* 246-275.

Eckert, E. A., D. Beard, and J. W. Beard. 1956. Virus of avian erythroblastosis. I. Titration of infectivity. J. Nat. Cancer Inst., *16:* 1099-1120.

Eckert, E. A., R. Rott, and W. Schäfer. 1964. Studies on the BAI strain A (avian myeloblastosis) virus. II. Some properties of viral split products. Virology, *24:* 434-440.

Ellermann, V. 1923. Histogenese der übertragbaren Huhnerleukose. IV. Zusammenfassende Betrachtungen. Folia Haematologia (Leipzig), *29:* 203-212.

Enders, J. F. 1964. Cell transformation by viruses as illustrated by the response of human and hamster renal cells to simian virus 40. The Harvey Lectures, *59:* 113-151.

Engelbreth-Holm, J. 1942. *Spontaneous and Experimental Leukemia in Animals.* Edinburgh: Oliver and Boyd.

Engelbreth-Holm, J., and A. Rothe-Meyer. 1935. On the connection between erythroblastosis (haemocytoblastosis), myelosis and sarcoma in chicken. Acta Path. Micro. Scand., *12:* 352-365.

Feldman, W. H., and C. Olson. 1965. Neoplastic disease of the chicken. In *Diseases of Poultry*, 5th ed., H. E. Biester and L. H. Schwartz, eds., pp. 863-924. Ames: Iowa State University Press.

Frederickson, T. N., H. G. Purchase, and B. R. Burmester. 1964. Transmission of virus from field cases of avian lymphomatosis. III. Variation in the oncogenic spectra of passaged virus isolates. Nat. Cancer Inst. Mono., *17:* 1-29.

Furth, J. 1933. Lymphomatosis, myelomatosis, and endothelioma of chickens caused by a filterable agent. I. Transmission experiments. J. Exp. Med., *58:* 253-275.

Furth, J. 1934. Lymphomatosis, myelomatosis, and endothelioma of chickens caused by a filterable agent. II. Morphological characteristics of the endotheliomata caused by this agent. J. Exp. Med., *59:* 501-517.

Gross, L. 1970. *Oncogenic Viruses*, 2nd ed. New York: Pergamon Press.

Gross, M. A., B. R. Burmester, and W. G. Walter. 1959. Pathogenicity of a viral strain (RPL 12) causing avian visceral lymphomatosis and related neoplasms. I. Nature of the lesions. J. Nat. Cancer Inst., 22: 83-101.

Hall, W. J., C. W. Bean, and M. Pollard. 1941. Transmission of fowl leukosis through chick embryos and young chicks. Am. J. Vet. Res., 2: 272-279.

Heine, U., G. de Thé, H. Ishiguro, J. R. Summer, D. Beard, and J. W. Beard. 1962. Multiplicity of cell response to the BAI strain A (myeloblastosis) avian tumor virus. II. Nephroblastoma (Wilms' tumor): Ultrastructure. J. Nat. Cancer Inst., 29: 41-105.

Heine, U., Z. Mladenov, D. Beard, and J. W. Beard. 1966. Morphology of hepatoma induced by strain MC29 avian leukosis virus. In Program of the 24th Ann. Meeting of the Electron Microscopy Society of America. B-21.

Hillman, E. A. 1971. Response of the liver to the avian leukosis agent, MC 29: A morphological study. Ph.D. dissertation, Duke University, Durham.

Ishiguro, H., D. Beard, J. R. Sommer, U. Heine, G. de Thé, and J. W. Beard. 1962. Multiplicity of cell response to the BAI strain A (myeloblastosis) avian tumor virus. I. Nephroblastoma (Wilms' tumor): Gross and microscopic pathology. J. Nat. Cancer Inst., 29: 1-39.

Ishizaki, R., and P. K. Vogt. 1966. Immunological relationships among envelope antigens of avian tumor viruses. Virology, 30: 375-387.

Ivanov, X., Z. Mladenov, S. Nedyalkov, T. G. Todorov, and M. Yakomov. 1964. Experimental investigations into avian leukosis. V. Transmission, haematology and morphology of avian myelocytomatosis. Bull. Inst. Path. Comp. Animaux, 10: 5-38.

Johnson, E. P. 1941. Fowl leukosis—manifestations, transmission, and etiological relationship of various forms. Virginia Agric. Expt. Sta. Tech. Bull. No. 76, pp. 3-21.

Langlois, A. J., and J. W. Beard. 1967. Converted-cell focus formation in culture by strain MC29 avian leukosis virus. Proc. Soc. Exp. Biol. Med., 126: 718-722.

Langlois, A. J., R. B. Fritz, U. Heine, D. Beard, D. P. Bolognesi, and J. W. Beard. 1969. Response of bone marrow to MC29 avian leukosis virus in vitro. Cancer Res., 29: 2056-2074.

Langlois, A. J., S. Sankaran, P. L. Hsiung, and J. W. Beard. 1967. Massive direct conversion of chick embryo cells by strain MC29 avian leukosis virus. J. Virol., 1: 1082-1084.

Langlois, A. J., L. Veprek, D. Beard, R. B. Fritz, and J. W. Beard. 1971. Isolation of a non-focus-forming agent from strain MC29 avian leukosis virus. Cancer Res., 31: 1010-1018.

Löliger, H. Ch. 1964. Histogenetic correlations between the reticular tissue and the different types of avian leukosis and related neoplasms. Nat. Cancer Inst. Mono., 17: 37-61.

Lucas, L., D. Beard, A. J. Langlois, and J. W. Beard. 1966. Strain ES4 avian leukosis virus: Titration and immunologic characterization. J. Immunol., 96: 85-95.

Mladenov, Z., U. Heine, D. Beard, and J. W. Beard. 1967. Strain MC29 avian leukosis virus. Myelocytoma, endothelioma, and renal growths: Pathomorphological and ultrastructural aspects. J. Nat. Cancer Inst., 38: 251-285.

Morgan, H. R., and W. Traub. 1964. Origin of Rous sarcoma strains. Nat. Cancer Inst. Mono., *17*: 392-393.

Olson, C., Jr. 1940. Transmissible fowl leukosis. A review of the literature. Mass. Agric. Expt. Sta. Bull. No. 370, pp. 1-48.

Olson, C., Jr. 1941. A transmissible lymphoid tumor of the chicken. Cancer Res., *1*: 384-392.

Purchase, H. G., and B. R. Burmester. 1972. Neoplastic Diseases: Leukosis-sarcoma group. In *Diseases of Poultry*, 6th ed., M. S. Hofsted, B. W. Calnek, C. F. Humbolt, W. M. Reid, and M. W. Yoder, Jr., eds., pp. 502-568. Ames: Iowa State University Press.

Rabotti, G. F., A. S. Grove, R. L. Sellers, and W. R. Anderson. 1966. Induction of multiple brain tumors (gliomata and leptomeningeal sarcomata) in dogs by Rous sarcoma virus. Nature (London), *209*: 884-886.

Rous, P. 1935. The virus tumors and the tumor problem. The Harvey Lectures, *31*: 74-115.

Sarma, P. S., H. C. Turner, and R. J. Huebner. 1964. An avian leukosis group-specific complement fixation reaction. Application for the detection and assay of non-cytopathogenic leukosis viruses. Virology, *23*: 313-321.

Stewart, H. L., and K. C. Snell. 1957. The histopathology of experimental tumors of the liver of the rat. A critical review of the histopathogenesis. Acta Un. Int. Cancer, *13*: 770-803.

Tozawa, H., H. Bauer, T. Graf, and H. Gelderblom. 1970. Strain-specific antigen of the avian leukosis sarcoma virus group. I. Isolation and immunological characterization. Virology, *40*: 530-539.

Veprek, L., D. Beard, A. J. Langlois, R. Ishizaki, and J. W. Beard. 1971. Transmission of avian myeloblastosis by BAI strain A virus ribonucleic acid. J. Nat. Cancer Inst., *46*: 713-729.

Vogel, K., W. Wittman, and K. Krieg. 1969. Virusbedingte Neoplasmen der Vögel (Virusbedingte avaire Tumoren). In *Handbuch der Virusinfektionen bei Tieren*, vol. 5, pp. 333-673. H. R. H. Ohrer, ed. Jena: Gustav Fischer Verlag.

Vogt, P. K. 1965. Avian tumor viruses. In *Advances in Virus Research*, vol. 11, pp. 293-385. K. M. Smith and M. A. Lauffer, eds. New York: Academic Press.

Vogt, P. K. 1969. Envelope classification of avian RNA tumor viruses. In *Comparative Leukemia Research*, R. M. Dutcher, ed., pp. 153-167. (*Bibl. haemat.* no. 36). Basel: S. Karger, 1970.

Structural Components of RNA Tumor Viruses

DANI P. BOLOGNESI, THOMAS RAINEY, and GUDRUN HÜPER
Department of Surgery, Duke University Medical Center
Durham, North Carolina

INTRODUCTION

AVIAN AND MAMMALIAN C-type RNA virus particles have many properties in common. They are assembled at the periphery of the host cell and elaborated by a process of budding such that the envelopment of the particles is achieved through acquisition of the host cell outer membrane (de Thé et al., 1964). Since throughout this process the interior of the budding particle is continuous with the cytoplasm, host constituents in this region of the cell could easily be incorporated into the virus. Indeed, the particles consist of several components of host cell origin and these will be discussed below.

Mature C-type viruses appear as spherical particles consisting of an outer bi-layered membrane and an inner concentrically localized core. Recent studies with Friend mouse leukemia virus suggest that the particle is, in fact, not a sphere but more closely resembles an icosahedron (Nermut et al., 1972). Measurements of the outer diameter of the particle vary from 80 to 140 nm, depending upon the virus preparation and the methods employed for fixation and staining.

Except in immature forms, the core component consists of a hexagonal inner shell which houses an electron-dense nucleoid. The diameter of the isolated avian virus core is between 75 nm and 85 nm (Bader et al., 1970; Bolognesi et al., 1972a; Gelderblom et al., 1972a; Stromberg, 1972), and that of the mammalian tumor virus core is similar (74 to 80 nm) (Luftig and Kilham, 1971; Nermut et al., 1972). Capsomere-like bodies have been visualized on the outer surface of the inner core shell of both avian and mammalian viruses (Bolognesi et al., 1972b; Gelderblom et al., 1972a; Nermut et al., 1972; Lange et al., 1973). The inner nucleoid most likely represents the virus RNA associated with protein. Suitable preparations of particles or cores have revealed a distinctly stranded nature of this material (Luftig and Kilham, 1971; Nermut et al., 1972). Electron microscopic evidence supports the view that both the core shell and the nucleoid are assembled at the bud site rather than being preformed elsewhere in the cell (de Thé et al., 1964).

Avian viruses reveal distinct projections on their outer surface (Bonar et al., 1963; Eckert et al., 1963). These components are visualized as a knoblike protrusion 6 nm in diameter connected to the virus surface by a thin spike 4 nm in length (Gelderblom et al., 1972a). The knob and spike project outward from the surface a distance of about 7 nm. They are strongly reminiscent of the surface hemagglutinin components of influenza viruses (Laver and Valentine, 1970). Biologically these materials represent the type-specific determinant of the virus (Tozawa et al., 1970; Duesberg et al., 1970; Bolognesi et al., 1972a), which is instrumental in distinguishing the various strains from one another (Vogt and Ishizaki, 1965, 1966; Ishizaki and Vogt, 1966). Similar structures on mammalian virus particles are much more difficult to visualize, and it has been suggested that they do not exist (Nowinski et al., 1970). However, recent work utilizing freeze-etching techniques has demonstrated clearly the presence of surface projections on Friend leukemia virus (Nermut et al., 1972; Witter et al., 1973). The surface projections of avian viruses also can be detected in discrete patches on the infected cell surface and concentrated in areas where virus particle maturation occurs (Gelderblom et al., 1972b). They are not found on normal cell surfaces (Gelderblom et al., 1972b).

I. AVIAN RNA TUMOR VIRUSES

By comparison to other mammalian viruses, the RNA tumor viruses are the most elaborate particles studied thus far. The avian myeloblastosis virus (AMV), a member of the chicken leukosis sarcoma group (ChiLSV) is representative of the avian agents and has been examined in most detail.

Chemical analysis of AMV indicated that the particles consist of 60 to 65 percent protein (Bonar and Beard, 1959), of which 5 to 7 percent is represented by glycoprotein. Approximately 30 to 35 percent of the dry weight of the virus is lipid, a large portion of which is phospholipid (Bonar and Beard, 1959; Rao et al., 1966; Quigley et al., 1971, 1972a). Ribonucleic acid constitutes about 2 percent of the dry weight of the particle (Bonar and Beard, 1959), and deoxyribonucleic acid about 0.04 percent (Levinson et al., 1972). Polysaccharides are present both in glycoproteins (Duesberg et al., 1970; Bolognesi and Bauer, 1970) and glycolipids (Quigley et al., 1971, 1972a). It is not known whether these measurements apply to all avian strains or how accurately they represent the composition of mammalian viruses. Certainly, the host cell from which the virus is derived has a great deal to do with the virus composition, particularly in regard to the lipid and polysaccharide moieties.

Purified virus particles consist of at least 17 polypeptides, on the basis of sodium dodecyl sulfate (SDS) gel electrophoresis, several of which have been identified in terms of their serological and structural properties. At least two of these are glycoproteins. Among the proteins, five distinct classes of enzymatic activities have been reported which include nucleic acid and protein synthesizing enzymes.

In terms of nucleic acids, five size classes of RNA are present in the particle. The largest component (60 to 70S) represents the virus genome and possesses an interesting segmented substructure. Each particle also contains 27S and 17S ribosomal RNA and transfer RNA. A small amount of RNA sedimenting at 7 to 9S is also present. Recently, various nucleotides also were reported to be present in the particle.

Proteins and Glycoproteins

The group-specific antigens

The basis for much of the work concerning the structural proteins of ChiLSV was the discovery of two distinct classes of antigenic activities associated with the virus particles. The first of these, located in the interior, is common to all members of the avian leukosis sarcoma complex and has, therefore, been referred to as the group-specific (gs) antigen of the virus (Huebner et al., 1964; Bauer and Schäfer, 1965). The second component, representing the strain-specific antigen of the virus (Vogt and Ishizaki, 1965; 1966; Ishizaki and Vogt, 1966), is situated on the outer surface of the virion (Rifkin and Compans, 1971; Bolognesi et al., 1972a).

For a long while, the *gs* component was considered as a single antigen (Bauer and Schäfer, 1966; Kelloff and Vogt, 1966; Payne et al., 1966; Allen, 1968, 1969). The work of Duesberg and co-workers (1968), however, demonstrated that following extraction of the virus with phenol and SDS and electrophoresis of the proteins in polyacrylamide gels, two major components could be distinguished which reacted with *gs* antisera. Multiple *gs* antigen components also were suggested by analyses of disrupted virus preparations in agar gel diffusion (Berman and Sarma, 1965; Roth and Dougherty, 1969; Armstrong, 1969).

This question was examined in some detail by analyses of large quantities of avian myeloblastosis virus (AMV) (Bolognesi and Bauer, 1970; Bauer and Bolognesi, 1970). Large-scale isolation of Rous sarcoma virus (RSV) polypeptides was also achieved by isoelectric focusing (Hung et al., 1971). Four major protein components were isolated by preparative acrylamide gel electrophoresis and analyzed for antigenicity (Bauer and Bolognesi, 1970). All four components reacted in complement fixation with *gs* antisera. Agar gel diffusion tests indicated that these materials were immunologically distinct. This work was extended and given a new dimension by Fleissner (1971). In this study, guanidine hydrochloride (Gu · HCl) chromatography on agarose columns was used to separate the virus polypeptides. This technique separates proteins on the basis of molecular weight and is particularly effective for low molecular weight proteins (Fish et al., 1969; Tung and Knight, 1972a,b). An excellent separation was obtained for the major virus polypeptides, and an additional protein component was resolved which co-electrophoresed with the most rapidly migrating polypeptide in SDS gel electrophoresis (Table 1). The proteins can be easily renatured following chromatography and appear to retain the major portion of their antigenicity (Fleissner, 1971; Bolognesi et al., 1973).

Previously it could not be determined with certainty whether or not all of the major virus proteins were group specific. Considerable evidence has been obtained that P5 (28,000 daltons) has all of the properties of a *gs* antigen. Although all of the virus strains tested contain very similar protein components as resolved on SDS or urea polyacrylamide electrophoresis, there is a detectable difference in the

Table 1. Avian myeloblastosis virus polypeptides

Polypeptide	Molecular weight (Gu · HCl)	Molecular weight (SDS)	Amino terminal group
P1	10,000	13,000	Valine
P2	12,000	15,000	Alanine
P3	15,000	13,000	Leucine
P4	19,000	23,000	ND
P5	27,000	28,000	Proline

proportion of the individual components from strain to strain (Bolognesi et al., 1974). It has not been ruled out that certain components might be subgroup specific. We have, therefore, compared the antigenicities of polypeptides isolated from two distinct virus strains —AMV (mainly subgroup B but traces of subgroup A) and Prague Rous sarcoma virus (entirely subgroup C). Our results (Bolognesi et al., 1973) indicate clearly that there is almost complete cross-reactivity among the individual gs antigens of the two viruses.

The type-specific antigens

An antigen on the surface of the virus presumably determines three distinct biological properties of ChiLSV; namely, the host range, the capacity to interfere with the infection of homologous but not with heterologous strains, and the induction of neutralizing antibody (Vogt and Ishizaki, 1965, 1966; Ishizaki and Vogt, 1966). The exact nature of this antigen remained in doubt for some time since the virus envelope contains a variety of components, many of which are derived from the host cell (for review, see Bolognesi and Obara, 1970). Furthermore, the virus contains 35 percent lipid by dry weight (Bonar and Beard, 1959; Quigley et al., 1971, 1972a), the major portion of which most likely resides on the envelope. Nevertheless, the knoblike protrusions on the surface of the virus (Bonar et al., 1963; Eckert et al., 1963) were the most likely site for this antigen since structurally and logistically they were best suited for specific interaction with the cell surface.

The first successful attempt to obtain this antigen in soluble form was performed by Tozawa and co-workers (1970). This material, which could be distinguished from gs antigens by sedimentation analysis, demonstrated all of the properties of the strain-specific antigen of the virus and was designated as virus envelope (Ve) antigen. A similar component was isolated from RSV (Duesberg et al., 1970) which consisted of two glycoproteins by gel electrophoretic analysis. The molecular weight of the major glycoprotein varied, depending on the strain used, and was in the region of 100,000 daltons; that of the minor component was about 37,000 daltons. Disruption of RSV with Brij 35, urea, and mercaptoethanol also released a complex containing the glycoproteins (Hung et al., 1971). Digestion of RSV with proteolytic enzymes under controlled conditions resulted in the removal of the glycoproteins from the outer surface (Rifkin and Compans, 1972) with loss of infectivity of the agent.

Sedimentation of AMV through a layer of nonionic detergent, Nonidet P40 (NP-40), made it possible to recover the virus envelope antigen quantitatively and in highly purified form as a material with interesting structural properties (Bolognesi et al., 1972a), (see below). This material consisted of about 7 percent of the protein and 60 percent of the carbohydrate content of the virus and was represented exclusively by the two virus glycoproteins.

Both glycoproteins specifically absorbed neutralizing sera and precipitated with these in immunodiffusion analysis, suggesting that each was involved in biological functions. In addition to the type-specific components, two distinct antigenic determinants were demonstrated by utilizing non-neutralizing sera (Bolognesi et al., 1972a). These determinants may represent surface subgroup-specific antigens previously suggested by Bauer and Graf (1969).

It is not certain which moiety of the glycoproteins is the type-specific antigenic determinant. Also, it is not known whether the carbohydrate portions are specified by the cell or by the virus. It is very difficult to remove the polysaccharides without destroying the proteins. Glycopeptides, however, can be recovered by proteolytic digestion of the protein (Lai and Duesberg, 1972). Such studies failed to reveal strain or subgroup-specific differences based on molecular weight of the glycopeptides. However, it was found that the glycopeptides of all viruses released from transformed cells were larger than those of viruses released from nontransformed cells. This suggests that the host cell plays a role in the formation of the polysaccharide components of AMV. Since this study measured the total glycopeptides of the virus, it is still not clear which of the glycopeptides are responsible for the differences. The glycoproteins represent only 60 percent of the virus polysaccharide content and it is not known where the remainder is located.

Arrangement in the Particle Structure

Although the morphological properties of ChiLSV have been well described, investigations of the relationship between the individual protein and nucleic acid constituents and the structural subunits of the agent have been initiated only recently. Specific identification of the virus substructures in terms of RNA and polypeptides is largely incomplete, but methods have been developed for homogeneous isolation of at least two major virus subunits—the outer envelope and the inner core. These materials have been analyzed by various means and the results provide some insight into the structural composition of the virus.

The virus surface

Components of the outer virus membrane are in part derived from the host cell as a direct consequence of the budding process of the particle (de Thé et al., 1964). Protruding from the membrane are distinct projections visualized as thin spikes with a knoblike component at their outer extremity (Bonar et al., 1963; Eckert et al., 1963). Treatment of RSV with bromelin under appropriate conditions results in the complete removal of the spike-knob projections, leaving a "naked" particle which has lost most of its biological infectivity (Rifkin and Campans, 1971).

Treatment of AMV with NP-40 releases the surface projections in a distinct aggregate which can be separated completely from other virus material by density gradient centrifugation (Bolognesi et al., 1972a). The free ends of the spike portions seem to aggregate end to end, as the spokes in a wheel, with the knobs remaining attached to the outer ends. This rosette-like structure measures 30 nm in diameter and sediments at about 33S. From its physical properties and electron microscopic appearance, it seems to be represented by an aggregate of about 12 surface projections. Similar structures have been observed following aggregation of the surface hemagglutinin and neuraminidase subunits of influenza viruses (Laver and Valentine, 1970).

Biologically, the rosettes represent the type-specific antigen of the virus. Biochemically, they consist of two virus glycoproteins, G1 (37,000 daltons) and G2 (100,000 daltons). Glycoprotein G2 makes up the knob and G1 the spike portions of the surface projections.

In addition to the type-specific (Ve) antigens, ChiLSV contain a second antigenic determinant on the surface membrane (Vm) (Ishizaki et al., 1973). Electron microscopic analysis of this material indicate the presence of a component resembling the outer membrane of the particle. Serological studies suggest that the outer membranes of ChiLSV are formed mainly from host cellular material.

An additional component located at or near the surface of the particle may be P1, as evidenced by surface-labeling studies (Bolognesi et al., 1973). Recent studies have shown that this material is associated with small amounts of carbohydrate.

The virus core

The following designations are proposed for the identification of the interior components of mature C-type virions:

1. *Core:* the entire inner substructure, representing nucleoid bordered by the core shell and capsomeres.

2. *Capsomeres:* hexagonally arranged subunits located on the surface of the core shell.

3. *Core shell:* the intermediate membrane of the virus enclosing the nucleoid.

4. *Nucleoid:* the innermost electron-dense material of the particle, consisting of the virus nucleic acid and associated proteins.

Initial attempts to quantitatively recover cores from avian RNA tumor viruses met with little success (Bonar et al., 1964; Duesberg, 1970). Some improvement was reported in a study by Bader and co-workers (1970), but neither the yields nor the homogeneity of the materials were adequate for meaningful analysis.

When milder conditions were used to disrupt the virus, structures resembling the virus core were obtained (Bolognesi et al., 1972b). The material banded at density of 1.25 g/cm³ in sucrose gradients, contained HMW RNA, reverse transcriptase, and the major group-specific antigen (P5). The core preparations were found to be infectious for chick embryo fibroblasts.

Unfortunately, the procedure used in these studies required a brief treatment with cold ether to prevent the cores from being trapped by lipid micelles formed after disruption of the virus with NP-40. This treatment may have been responsible for the removal or loss of certain core constituents (see below).

A more suitable procedure for core isolation was described by Stromberg (1972). Treatment of AMV with the surfactant, Sterox

SL, gave rise to quantitative yields of homogeneous virus cores. They, too, banded at a density of 1.26 g/cm³ in sucrose gradients.

Other workers, concerned with the isolation of internal virion components, have observed an apparently different structure. Treatment of RSV with Triton X (Coffin and Temin, 1971; Davis and Rueckert, 1972) or NP-40 (Quigley et al., 1972b) released a material which resembled the inner nucleoid component. Its density is somewhat greater than that of cores; 1.36 in D₂O-sucrose (Davis and Rueckert, 1972) or 1.27 to 1.29 in sucrose (Quigley et al., 1972b; Smith, unpub.). These subunits consist of most of the virion HMW RNA (Davis and Rueckert, 1972) associated with several protein components, the major one being P2. Forty percent of the 4S RNA also was associated with this structure, as was reverse transcriptase activity (Davis and Rueckert, 1972). These "ribonucleoprotein particles" seem to lack phospholipid or glucosamine, consist of about 20 percent RNA and 80 percent protein, and possess a sedimentation coefficient of about 130S (Davis and Rueckert, 1972).

Work in our laboratory employing newer procedures to isolate virus particle cores in high quality preparations from various strains of avian tumor agents (Bolognesi et al., 1973) has helped correlate the studies cited above. Recent results indicate that the cores used in our earlier studies (Bolognesi et al., 1972b) lacked several protein components in spite of a strong similarity in structure.

Sedimentation of AMV through layers of the surfactant Sterox SL and the nonionic detergent NP-40 and then to equilibrium in a sucrose gradient gave rise to a homogeneous preparation of cores at a density of 1.26 g/cm³ (Bolognesi et al., 1973). Analysis of such preparations for polypeptide content revealed (Fig. 1) that two of the five major virus proteins, P5 and P2, are present in large quantity, while P3 is present in a much lower quantity. This latter polypeptide was identified by chromatography of the core material in guanidine hydrochloride or by electrophoresis in a urea-acrylamide system at neutral pH. Several minor components are also present, most notable being a polypeptide of about 37,000 molecular weight (P6). This component, whose migration property is similar to that of G1, does not appear to be a glycoprotein.

By further disruption of the isolated cores, a complex consisting of virus RNA, reverse transcriptase, and polypeptide P2 was isolated (Fig. 1). This material has a density greater than 1.30 g/cm³ in sucrose and under electron microscopy resembles the internal

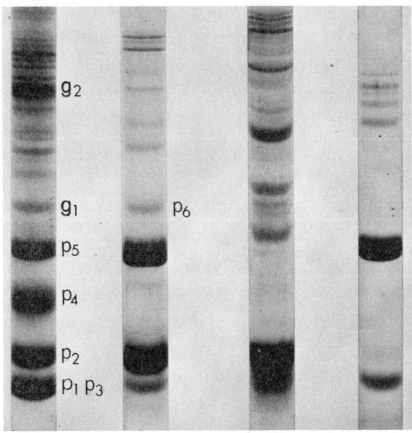

Figure 1.   Polypeptide composition of AMV subviral components. From left to right: AMV; AMV cores; AMV RNP; top of AMV RNP gradient. The material migrating below AMV P2 in the RNP gradient is not AMV P3 since essentially all of P3 can be found at the top of the RNP gradient. An almost complete recovery of the core polypeptides was achieved in these two fractions. The RNP material, probably because of the way it was isolated, has repeatedly been difficult to fractionate in our SDS gel system. The curvature of the bands, and possibly their number (some may be aggregates), indicates this.

nucleoid component. At the top of this gradient, the remainder of the major core polypeptides (P5 and P3) are present in a homogeneous band. Electron microscopic analysis has suggested the presence of fragments of the core shell. These findings suggest that the major polypeptides P5 and P3 are associated with the core shell, while P2 is closely associated with the RNA. Polypeptide analysis of the top fractions of the gradient reveals the presence of the missing core components (Fig. 2).

A model for the avian myeloblastosis virus is presented in Figure 3. The basis for the localization of the various components is derived from published data, manuscripts in press, and unpublished observations in this and other laboratories. Not all of the virus substructures can be identified with certainty in terms of polypeptide composition at the present time. The two virus glycoproteins (G1 and G2) and P1 appear to be associated with the virus envelope on

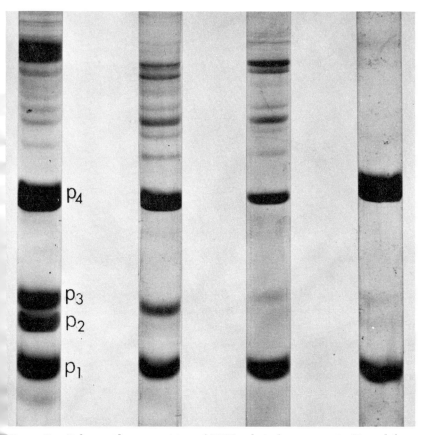

Figure 2.   Polypeptide composition of FLV subviral components. From left to right: FLV; FLV cores; FLV RNP; top of FLV RNP gradient. A complete separation of the surface components of the core and those in the RNP material was apparently not achieved, in contrast to the situation in AMV (see Fig. 1, text).

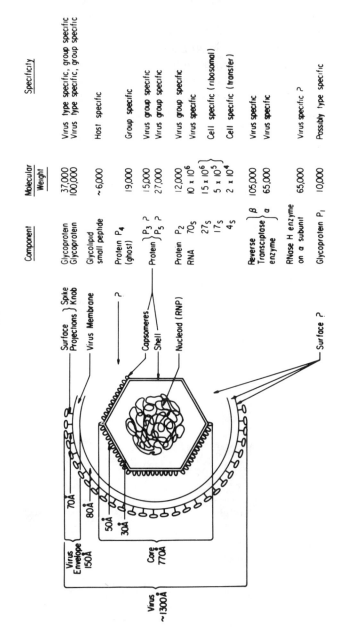

STRUCTURAL COMPONENTS OF AMV

	Component	Molecular Weight	Specificity
Surface Projections } Spike / Knob	Glycoprotein / Glycoprotein	37,000 / 100,000	Virus type specific, group specific / Virus type specific, group specific
Virus Membrane	Glycolipid small peptide	~6,000	Host specific
?	Protein P$_4$ (ghost)	19,000	Group specific
Capsomeres	Protein } P$_3$? } P$_5$?	15,000 / 27,000	Virus group specific / Virus group specific
Shell	Protein P$_2$	12,000	Virus group specific
Nucleoid (RNP)	RNA 70s	10 x 10^6	Virus specific
	27s	15 x 10^6	Cell specific (ribosomal)
	17s	5 x 10^5	
	4s	2 x 10^4	Cell specific (transfer)
	Reverse Transcriptase enzyme } β / α	105,000 / 65,000	Virus specific / Virus specific
	RNase H enzyme on α subunit	65,000	Virus specific ?
Surface ?	Glycoprotein P$_1$	10,000	Possibly type specific

Virus Envelope 150Å — 70Å, 80Å, 50Å, 30Å

Core 770Å

Virus ~1300Å

Figure 3. Model of the avian myeloblastosis virus particle (AMV). Structurally, the model is essentially that of Gelderblom and co-workers (1972a) and is representative of avian C-type viruses. The basis for the localization of the various components is discussed in the text. As indicated in the diagram, most of the virus nucleic acids and associated enzymes are localized in the nucleoid of the particle.

the basis of surface-labeling studies (Bolognesi et al., 1975). In addition to carbohydrate and lipid, isolated virus surface membranes (Vm) contain a low molecular weight polypeptide whose origin is unclear (Ishizaki et al., 1973). Polypeptides P3 and P5 (Fig. 1) are not contained in the nucleoid (RNP). Therefore, they probably are associated with the core surface. However, the low recovery of P3 (10-15%) in core preparations does not permit a definitive conclusion for the localization of this protein thus far. Polypeptide P4, the ghost protein, has not been localized, but it seems clear that it is neither an outer envelope nor a core component.

The nucleoid of the particle is apparently very complex. As indicated in Figure 1, it contains several HMW polypeptides in addition to the basic protein, P2. Some of these may represent the various enzyme activities in the virus, particularly the reverse transcriptase, RNase H, and other related enzymes. All of these appear to be somehow associated with the virus RNA. The entire complex has a density greater than 1.30 g/cm^3, a sedimentation constant of about 130S, and some structural definition (see above).

In addition to the 70S RNA, minor ribosomal RNA components can be detected in the core (Bolognesi et al., 1971, 1972b). Recent evidence shows that a substantial portion of the virion transfer RNA can be found in cores (Stromberg and Litwak, 1973). This is not inconsistent with previous work where only a small proportion of low molecular weight RNA was present in the core, since the transfer RNA represents only 25 percent of the virion 4S RNA (Bonar et al., 1967).

II. MAMMALIAN RNA TUMOR VIRUSES

The principal avian RNA tumor viruses are those which belong to the chicken leukosis-sarcoma complex. Not until recently has there been any concrete evidence that similar viruses exist in other avian species (Hanafusa and Hanafusa, 1973). This differs from the situation with mammalian RNA tumor viruses. Agents belonging to the C-type class have been isolated from at least eight different mammalian species. Those isolated from mice and cats have been studied extensively, and a great deal of information is being accumulated for the other viruses.

The various C-type agents found in mammals are similar in structure and composition as regards their major constituents such as nucleic acids, proteins, and enzymes. As indicated above, they have a remarkable similarity in these respects to the avian agents. However, distinct differences in the serological properties of the major virus proteins together with specificity of the virus reverse transcriptases have served effectively to identify and characterize viruses isolated from different species and to differentiate other families or classes of virions.

Proteins and Glycoproteins

Analysis of mammalian RNA tumor virus polypeptides by SDS gel electrophoresis reveals, in most cases, three major and several minor components (Gilden et al., 1971; Schäfer et al., 1971; Oroszlan et al., 1971; Moroni, 1972; Schäfer et al., 1972; Oroszlan et al., 1972a, b) (Fig. 2). The pattern is distinctly different from that of avian viruses, which have four polypeptides in roughly similar amounts (see Fig. 1). However, as with the avian viruses, gel filtration in guanidine hydrochloride (Gu · HCl) resolves a component which is not distinguishable by electrophoresis in SDS-containing gels (Nowinski et al., 1972). This material co-electrophoreses with the second most rapidly migrating component in the gel and its molecular weight in guanidine hydrochloride is about 10,000 daltons (Green and Bolognesi, 1974).

The molecular weights of the major polypeptides of Friend leukemia virus (FLV) and the Rickard strain of feline leukemia virus (FeLV) are indicated in Table 2. The values, which are nearly identical for the two viruses, correspond to those reported for other C-type mammalian oncornaviruses by Nowinski and co-workers (1972) using a similar method, but differ somewhat with those estimated by SDS gel electrophoresis (Gilden et al., 1971; Moroni, 1972; Schäfer et al., 1971, 1972). As indicated above, the molecular weights obtained by gel filtration in Gu · HCl are considered to be more accurate, since this method has proven more reliable for polypeptides in this molecular weight range (Fish et al., 1971; Tung and Knight, 1972a,b).

The status of glycoproteins in the mammalian viruses is not as well defined as in avian viruses. Material which incorporates radioactively labeled glucosamine or stains for carbohydrate on analysis with SDS gel electrophoresis indicates the presence of two or more

Table 2.   Polypeptides of Friend leukemia virus (FLV) and feline leukemia
virus (FeLV)

Polypeptide	Molecular Weight (Gu · HCl)
P1	10,000
P2	12,000
P3	15,000
P4	31,000

glycoproteins in the high molecular weight region of the gel (Duesberg et al., 1970; Moroni, 1972; Schäfer et al., 1972; Witter et al.,
1973). The major glycoprotein component has an estimated molecular weight of 60,000 to 80,000 daltons, and the minor between 40,000
to 50,000 daltons. Initially, it was not certain that these glycoproteins
corresponded to the components of the surface projections of the
virion, as is the case for avian viruses. However, studies by Duesberg and co-workers (1970) indicate that this is most probable (Fig.
4). Recently, Witter and co-workers (1973a,b) have concluded that
the surface projections not only correspond the to the glycoproteins,
but that they also represent the hemagglutinin component of these
viruses.

Studies in this laboratory indicate that, in addition to the HMW
glycoproteins, component p2 is associated with about 5 percent
carbohydrate, very little of which is glucosamine. This component
stains red with Coomassie blue and appears to be analogous to
avian P1.

Some work has been reported on the amino acid composition
(Schäfer et al., 1969) and N-terminal amino acid sequences of the
major polypeptide of various mammalian oncornaviruses (Oroszlan
et al., 1972c). The latter studies indicate that the N-terminal sequences of avian P5 and murine p4 are distinctly different. On the
other hand, the first three residues of p4 from murine and feline
agents are identical. Much more needs to be done, however, to es-
tablish the extent of homology of the corresponding components of
viruses from related and unrelated species origin.

Single amino acid labeling studies suggest that of the four
major polypeptides, component p1 is rich in arginine (Moroni, 1972;
Bolognesi, unpub.). Direct amino acid analyses of polypeptides from
mouse and feline leukemia viruses in this laboratory support the
notion that p1 is the most basic protein in the virus.

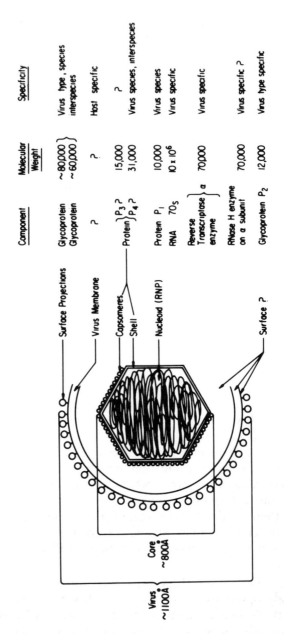

Figure 4.   Model of the Friend leukemia virus particle (FLV). The structural appearance and dimensions of this murine virus were taken from Nermut and co-workers (1972). In comparison to AMV (Fig. 3), much less is known about the composition of the subviral components.

Structural Aspects

The morphological properties of mammalian C-type viruses are quite similar to those of their avian counterparts. There are, however, distinct differences in certain aspects of their structure.

As pointed out earlier, the surface projections in mammalian viruses are not as prominent as those in avian viruses. A well-defined spike which attaches the knob to the virus surface is apparently lacking. The structure of the virus core and the inner nucleoid component appears also to differ from that of analogous components of avian viruses. Some authors suggest that the mammalian cores occupy a larger proportion of the virus interior than do the avian cores (Nermut et al., 1972; Gelderblom et al., 1972a) (see Figs. 3, 4). The capsomere arrangement on the mammalian core surface is much more distinct (Nermut et al., 1972) than what has been described for AMV cores (Bolognesi et al., 1972b; Gelderblom et al., 1972a). However, other authors have not detected capsomeres in association with mammalian cores (Sarkar et al., 1971; Luftig and Kilham, 1971). Some controversy exists also as to whether or not the core contains an outer shell (Sarkar et al., 1971), as reported by Nermut and co-workers (1972). Perhaps these discrepancies result from different techniques used to isolate and visualize the cores (Luftig and Kilham, 1971).

The internal electron-dense component of the mammalian virus core is composed of whorled strandlike material (Luftig and Kilham, 1971; Nermut et al., 1972) rather than a compact nucleoid as described for AMV (Bolognesi et al., 1972b; Gelderblom et al., 1972a) (see Figs. 3, 4). This inner component of mammalian virus cores seems to be closely associated with the core surface; in contrast, with AMV cores a "space" can be seen between the nucleoid and the core shell. Recent studies in which avian and mammalian virus cores were sectioned and examined in the electron microscope seem to confirm this observation (Bolognesi et al., 1973).

Localization of the C-type mammalian virion components in the particle structure is not as advanced as with avian agents. Nevertheless, some of these components can be identified on the basis of recent work.

As with avian viruses, the surface projections of FLV are represented by glycoproteins (Witter et al., 1973a,b); Moennig et al., 1974). It is of interest that an antigenic determinant with interspecies cross-reactivity also appears to be associated with the virion surface

(Witter et al., 1973a,b). Possibly the same material could be detected by gel precipitation or radioimmunoassay (Strand and August, 1973). Its molecular weight is about 70,000 daltons and it is distinct from the reverse transcriptase enzyme (Strand and August, 1973).

Polypeptide p2, which is associated with some carbohydrate (Bolognesi et al., 1973), may be a further surface component of the virion although this is not indicated by surface labeling studies using I^{25} (Witte et al., 1973). This may reflect the lack of available tyrosine sites on this component when it is situated on or in the virion surface. It is not known which, if any, of these glycoproteins correspond to the group-specific surface antigen of murine viruses described by Aoki and co-workers (1971).

Attempts to isolate mammalian virus cores in quantitative yields have been described (de Thé and O'Connor, 1966; Shibley et al., 1967), and it has been reported that such preparations possess biological activity (Rauscher, 1962; Shibley et al., 1967, 1969). Analysis of virion components in these materials, however, was not carried out. Recent work utilizing similar techniques (Lange et al., 1973) or procedures analogous to those used for isolation of avian cores (Bolognesi et al., 1973) have given rise to semiquantitative yields of homogeneous virus cores containing protein nucleic acid and reverse transcriptase activity. The major core polypeptides in each study were found to be p4 and p1 (Fig. 2). Enrichment of the basic protein, p1 (Fig. 2), could be obtained by further degradation of the cores to a material resembling the internal component of avian cores (see Fig. 1). However, these preparations contained a substantial amount of p4 (Fig. 2), suggesting that in contrast to the situation with avian viruses (see Fig. 1), the separation of the ribonucleoprotein particle from the core surface constituents was not complete. As suggested by the ultrastructural observations, this may reflect a closer association of the internal and surface constituents of mammalian virus cores. The model depicted in Figure 4, which is essentially that of Nermut and co-workers (1972) in terms of structure, illustrates the information discussed above.

CONCLUSION

The structural properties of C-type oncornaviruses have been summarized in the models presented in Figures 3 and 4. It appears that the avian and mammalian agents contain similar polypeptides

Table 3. Localization of major oncornavirus structural components

	Avian			Mammalian		
	Designation[1]		Site	Designation[1]		Site
Major polypeptides	P 1*	p 10	Virion surface	p 1	p 10	Core interior (RNP)
	P 2	p 12	Core interior (RNP)	p 2*	p 12	Virion surface
	P 3	p 15	Core surface (?)	p 3	p 15	Core surface (?)
	P 4	p 19	Virion interior			Absent
	P 5	p 27	Core surface	p 4	p 30	Core surface
Glycoproteins	G 1	gp 35	Surface spike	(G 1)	gp 45	Virion surface
	G 2	gp 85	Surface knob	(G 2)	gp 69/71	Virion carbohydrate

[1] Nomenclature used by Bolognesi in left-hand column; new nomenclature (August et al., 1974) in right-hand column.

* Designations marked with an asterisk are associated with carbohydrate.

in analogous structural components. The localization of the major components for each agent is illustrated in Table 3.

A great deal of information about these viruses, particularly their origin and relationship to one another, can be obtained by studying the structural components of the particles. Such information is necessary for the detection and identification of unknown viruses and for the analysis of structural components in the host cell. Utilizing various oncornavirus structural elements as reagents and tools, workers are searching for analogous materials in human malignant cells. Promising results have been obtained in several laboratories.

Acknowledgments: Preparation of this manuscript was aided by Research Contract NO1 CP 33308 from the Special Virus Cancer Program of the National Cancer Institute.

The authors are grateful to other members of the laboratory for their cooperation in this work. Dr. R. Green has carried out the isolation and purification of the virus polypeptides (Green and Bolognesi, 1974); Dr. R. Ishizaki has carried out the analyses of the virus surface membrane (Ishizaki et al., 1973); and Dr. A. J. Langlois has provided invaluable assistance in the development of necessary biological systems and the production of much of the virus used. We are indebted to Dr. R. Luftig of the Department of Microbiology for all of the electron microscopy, which has appeared in a separate publication (Bolognesi et al., 1973).

Literature Cited

Allen, D. W. 1968. Characterization of avian leukosis group-specific antigen from avian myeloblastosis. Biochim. Biophys. Acta, *154:* 388-396.

Allen, D. W. 1969. The N-terminal amino acid of an avian leukosis group-specific antigen from avian myeloblastosis virus. Virology, *38:* 32-41.

Aoki, T., P. A. Herberman, M. Johnson, M. Liu, and M. Sturm. 1971. Wild-type Gross leukemia virus: Classification of soluble antigens. J. Virol., *10:* 1208-1219.

Armstrong, D. 1969. Multiple group-specific antigen components of avian tumor viruses detected with chicken and hamster sera. J. Virol., *3:* 133-139.

August, J. T., D. P. Bolognesi, E. Fleissner, R. V. Gilden, and R. C. Nowinski. 1974. A proposed nomenclature for the virion proteins of oncogenic RNA viruses. Virology, *60:* 595-601.

Bader, J. P., N. R. Brown, and A. V. Bader. 1970. Characteristics of cores of avian leuko-sarcoma viruses. Virology, *41:* 718-728.

Bauer, H., and D. P. Bolognesi. 1970. Polypeptides of avian RNA tumor viruses. II. Biological characterization. Virology, *42:* 1113-1126.

Bauer, H., and T. Graf. 1969. Evidence for the existence of two envelope antigenic components and corresponding cell receptors for avian tumor viruses. Virology, *37:* 157-161.

Bauer, H., and W. Schäfer. 1966. Origin of group-specific antigen of chicken leukosis viruses. Virology, 29: 494-496.

Berman, L. D., and P. S. Sarma. 1965. Demonstration of an avian leukosis group antigen by immunodiffusion. Nature (London), 207: 263-265.

Bolognesi, D. P., and H. Bauer. 1970. Polypeptides of avian RNA tumor viruses. I. Isolation and physical and chemical analysis. Virology, 42: 1097-1112.

Bolognesi, D. P., H. Bauer, H. Gelderblom, and G. Hüper. 1972a. Polypeptides of avian RNA tumor viruses. IV. Components of the viral envelope. Virology, 47: 551-566.

Bolognesi, D. P., H. Bauer, H. Gelderblom, and K. Mölling. 1971. Structural components of avian myeloblastosis virus. In Unifying Concepts of Leukemia, R. M. Dutcher and L. Chieco-Bianchi, eds., pp. 316-360. (Bibl. haemat, no. 39). Basel: S. Karger, 1973.

Bolognesi, D. P., H. Gelderblom, H. Bauer, K. Mölling, and G. Hüper. 1972b. Polypeptides of avian tumor viruses. V. Analysis of the virus core. Virology, 47: 567-578.

Bolognesi, D. P., G. Hüper, R. W. Green, and T. Graf. 1974. Biochemical properties of oncornavirus polypeptides. Biochim. Biophys. Acta, Rev. on Cancer, 355: 220-235.

Bolognesi, D. P., R. Ishizaki, G. Hüper, T. C. Vanaman, and R. E. Smith, 1975. Immunological properties of avian oncornavirus polypeptides. Virology, 64: 349-357.

Bolognesi, D. P., R. Luftig, and J. H. Shaper. 1973. Localization of RNA tumor virus polypeptides. I. Isolation of further virus substructures. Virology, 56: 549-564.

Bolognesi, D. P., and T. Obara. 1969. Minor RNA and other components of host origin intrinsic to avian leukosis virus particles. In Comparative Leukemia Research, R. M. Dutcher, ed., pp. 126-139. (Bibl. haemat. no. 36). Basel: S. Karger, 1970.

Bonar, R. A., and J. W. Beard. 1959. Virus of avian myeloblastosis. XII. Chemical constitution. J. Nat. Cancer Inst., 23: 183-197.

Bonar, R. A., U. Heine, D. Beard, and J. W. Beard. 1963. Virus of avian myeloblastosis (BAI strain A). XXIII. Morphology of the virus and comparison with strain R (erythroblastosis). J. Nat. Cancer Inst., 30: 949-997.

Bonar, R. A., U. Heine, and J. W. Beard. 1964. Structure of BAI strain A (myeloblastosis) avian tumor virus. Nat. Cancer Inst. Mono., 17: 589-614.

Bonar, R. A., L. Sverak, D. P. Bolognesi, A. J. Langlois, D. Beard, and J. W. Beard. 1967. Ribonucleic acid components of BAI strain A (myeloblastosis) avian tumor virus. Cancer Res., 27: 1138-1157.

Coffin, J. M., and H. M. Temin. 1971. Comparison of Rous sarcoma virus-specific deoxyribonucleic acid polymerase in virions of Rous sarcoma virus-infected chicken cells. J. Virol., 7: 625-634.

Davis, N. L., and R. R. Rueckert. 1972. Properties of a ribonuc'eoprotein particle isolated from Nonidet P-40-treated Rous sarcoma virus. J. Virol., 10: 1010-1020.

de Thé, G., C. Becker, and J. W. Beard. 1964. Virus of avian myeloblastosis (BAI strain A): XXV. Ultracytochemical study of virus and myeloblast phosphatase activity. J. Nat. Cancer Inst., 32: 201-235.

de Thé, G., and T. E. O'Connor. 1966. Structure of a murine leukemia virus after disruption with Tween-ether and comparison with two myxoviruses. Virology, 28: 713-728.

Duesberg, P. H. 1970. On the structure of RNA tumor viruses. Curr. Top. Microbiol Immunol., 51: 79-104.

Duesberg, P. H., G. S. Martin, and P. K. Vogt. 1970. Glycoprotein components of avian and murine RNA tumor viruses. Virology, 41: 631-646.

Duesberg, P. H., H. L. Robinson, W. S. Robinson, R. J. Huebner, and H. C. Turner. 1968. Proteins of Rous sarcoma virus. Virology, 36: 68-73.

Eckert, E. A., R. Rott, and W. Schäfer. 1963. Myxovirus-like structure of avian myeloblastosis virus. Z. Naturforsch. B., 18: 339-340.

Fish, W., K. Mann, and C. Tanford. 1969. The estimation of polypeptide chain molecular weights by gel filtration in 6M guanidine hydrochloride. J. Biol. Chem., 244: 4989-4994.

Fleissner, E. 1971. Chromatographic separation and antigenic analysis of proteins of the oncornaviruses. I. Avian leukemia-sarcoma viruses. J. Virol., 8: 778-785.

Gelderblom, H., H. Bauer, D. P. Bolognesi, and H. Frank. 1972a. Morphogenese und Aufbau von RNA-Tumorviren: Elektronenoptische Untersuchungen an Virus-Partikeln vom C-Typ. Zbl. Bakt. Hyg., I. Abt. Orig. A., 220: 79-90.

Gelderblom, H., H. Bauer, and T. Graf. 1972b. Cell-surface antigens induced by avian RNA tumor viruses: Detection by immunoferritin technique. Virology 47: 416-425.

Gilden, R., S. Oroszlan, and R. Huebner. 1971. Coexistence of intraspecies and interspecies specific antigenic determinants on the major structural polypeptide of mammalian L-type viruses. Nature New Biol., 231: 107-108.

Green, R. W., and D. P. Bolognesi. 1974. Isolation of proteins by gel filtration in 6M guanidinium chloride: Applications to RNA tumor viruses. Anal. Biochem., 57: 108-117.

Hanafusa, T., and H. Hanafusa. 1973. Isolation of leukosis-type virus from pheasant embryo cells. Possible presence of viral genes in cells. Virology, 51: 247-251.

Herman, A. C., R. W. Green, D. P. Bolognesi, and T. C. Vanaman. 1975. Comparative chemical properties of avian oncornavirus polypeptides. Virology, 64: 339-348.

Huebner, R. J., D. Armstrong, M. Okuyan, P. S. Sarma, and H. C. Turner. 1964. Specific complement-fixing antigens in hamster and guinea pig tumors induced by Schmidt-Rippin strain of avian sarcoma. Proc. Nat. Acad. Sci. U.S., 51: 742-750.

Hung, P. H., H. L. Robinson, and W. S. Robinson. 1971. Isolation and characterization of proteins from Rous sarcoma virus. Virology, 43: 251-266.

Ishizaki, R., R. B. Luftig, and D. P. Bolognesi. 1973. Outer membrane of avian myeloblastosis virus. J. Virol., 12: 1579-1588.

Ishizaki, R., and P. K. Vogt. 1966. Immunological relationships among envelope antigens of avian tumor viruses. Virology, 30: 375-387.

Kelloff, G., and P. K. Vogt. 1966. Localization of avian tumor virus group-specific antigen in cell and virus. Virology, 29: 377-384.

Lai, M., and P. H. Duesberg. 1972. Differences between the envelope glyco-proteins and glycopeptides of avian tumor viruses released from trans-formed and from nontransformed cells. Virology, 50: 359-372.

Lange, J., H. Frank, G. Hunsmann, V. Moennig, R. Wollman, and W. Schäfer. 1973. Properties of mouse leukemia viruses. VI. The core of Friend virus: Isolation and constituents. Virology, 53: 457-462.

Laver, W. G., and R. C. Valentine. 1969. Morphology of the isolated hemag-glutinin and neuraminidase subunits of influenza virus. Virology, 38: 105-119.

Levinson, W. E., H. E. Varmus, A. C. Garapin, and J. M. Bishop. 1972. DNA of Rous sarcoma virus: Its nature and significance. Science, 175: 76-78.

Luftig, R. B., and S. S. Kilham. 1971. An electron microscope study of Rau-scher leukemia virus. Virology, 46: 277-297.

Moennig, V., H. Frank, G. Hunsmann, I. Schneider, and W. Schäfer. 1974. Properties of mouse leukemia viruses. VII. The major viral glycoproteins of Friend leukemia virus: Isolation and physicochemical properties. Vi-rology, 61: 100-111.

Moroni, C. 1972. Structural proteins of Rauscher leukemia virus and Harvey sarcoma virus. Virology, 47: 1-7.

Nermut, M. V., H. Frank, and W. Schäfer. 1972. Properties of mouse leukemia viruses. III. Electron microscopic appearance as revealed after conventional preparation techniques as well as freeze-drying and freeze-etching. Vi-rology, 49: 345-358.

Nowinski, R. C., E. Fleissner, N. Sarkar, and T. Aoki. 1972. Chromatographic separation and antigenic analysis of proteins of the oncornaviruses. II. Mammalian leukemia sarcoma viruses. J. Virol., 9: 359-366.

Nowinski, R. C., L. J. Old, N. H. Sarkar, and D. H. Moore. 1970. Common properties of the oncogenic RNA viruses (oncornaviruses). Virology, 42: 1152-1157.

Oroszlan, S., R. Bova, R. Huebner, and R. Gilden. 1972a. Major group-specific protein of rat type C viruses. J. Virol., 10: 746-750.

Oroszlan, S., R. Bova, M. White, R. Toni, C. Foreman, and R. Gilden. 1972b. Purification and immunological characterization of the major internal protein of the RD-114 virus. Proc. Nat. Acad. Sci. U.S., 69: 1211-1215.

Oroszlan, S., T. Copeland, M. Summers, and R. V. Gilden. 1972c. Amino termi-nal sequences of the mammalian type C RNA tumor virus group-specific antigens. Biochem. Biophys. Res. Commun., 48: 1549-1555.

Oroszlan, S., R. Huebner, and R. Gilden. 1971. Species-specific and inter-specific antigenic determinants associated with the structural protein of the feline C-type virus. Proc. Nat. Acad. Sci. U.S., 68: 901-904.

Payne, F. E., J. J. Solomon, and H. G. Purchase. 1966. Immunofluorescent studies of group-specific antigen of the avian sarcoma-leukemia viruses. Proc. Nat. Acad. Sci. U.S., 55: 341-348.

Quigley, J. P., D. B. Rifkin, and R. W. Compans. 1972a. Isolation and charac-terization of ribonucleoprotein substructures from Rous sarcoma virus. Virology, 50: 65-75.

Quigley, J. P., D. B. Rifkin, and E. Reich. 1971. Phospholipid composition of Rous sarcoma virus, host cell membranes and other enveloped RNA viruses. Virology, 46: 106-116.

Quigley, J. P., D. B. Rifkin, and E. Reich. 1972b. Lipid studies of Rous sarcoma virus and host cell membranes. Virology, 50: 550-557.

Rao, P. R., R. A. Bonar, and J. W. Beard. 1966. Lipids of the BAI strain A avian tumor virus and of the myeloblast host cells. Exp. Mol. Pathol., 5: 374-378.

Rauscher, F. J. 1962. A virus-induced disease of mice characterized by erythropoiesis and lymphoid leukemia. J. Nat. Cancer Inst., 29: 515-543.

Rifkin, D. B., and R. W. Compans. 1971. Identification of the spike proteins of Rous sarcoma virus. Virology, 46: 485-489.

Roth, F. K., and R. M. Dougherty. 1969. Multiple antigenic components of the group-specific antigen of the avian leukosis-sarcoma viruses. Virology, 38: 278-284.

Sarkar, N. H., R. C. Nowinski, and D. H. Moore. 1971. Helical nucleocapsid structure of the oncogenic ribonucleic acid viruses (oncornaviruses). J. Virol., 8: 564-572.

Schäfer, W., F. A. Anderer, H. Bauer, and L. Pister. 1969. Studies on mouse leukemia viruses. I. Isolation and characterization of a group-specific antigen. Virology, 38: 387-394.

Schäfer, W., J. Lange, D. P. Bolognesi, F. deNoronha, J. Post, and C. Rickard. 1971. Isolation and characterization of two group-specific antigens from feline leukemia virus. Virology, 44: 73-82.

Schäfer, W., J. Lange, P. J. Fischinger, H. Frank, D. P. Bolognesi, and L. Pister. 1972. Properties of mouse leukemia viruses. II. Isolation of viral components. Virology, 47: 210-228.

Shibley, G. P., F. J. Carleton, B.S. Wright, G. Shidlovsky, J. H. Monroe, and S. A. Mayyasi. 1969. Comparison of the biologic and biophysical properties of the progeny of intact and ether-extracted Rauscher leukemia viruses. Cancer Res., 29: 905-909.

Shibley, G. P., F. E. Durr, G. Shidlovsky, B. S. Wright, and R. Schmitter. 1967. Leukemogenic activity of ether-extracted Rauscher leukemia virus. Science, 156: 1610-1613.

Strand, M., and J. T. August. 1973. Structural proteins of oncogenic ribonucleic acid viruses. J. Biol. Chem., 248: 5627-5633.

Stromberg, K. 1972. Surface-active agents for isolation of the core component of avian myeloblastosis virus. J. Virol., 9: 684-697.

Stromberg, K., and M. D. Litwack. 1973. Structural studies of avian myeloblastosis virus: Presence of transfer RNA in core component. Biochim. Biophys. Acta, 319: 140-152.

Tozawa, H., H. Bauer, T. Graf, and H. Gelderblom. 1970. Strain-specific antigen of avian leukosis sarcoma group. I. Isolation and immunological characterization. Virology, 40: 530-539.

Tung, J.-S., and C. A. Knight. 1972a. Relative importance of some factors affecting the electrophoretic migration of proteins in sodium dodecylsulfate-polyacrylamide gels. Anal. Biochem., 48: 153-163.

Tung, J.-S., and C. A. Knight. 1972b. The coat protein subunits of cucumber viruses 3 and 4 and a comparison of methods for determining their molecular weights. Virology, 48: 574-581.

Vogt, P. K., and R. Ishizaki. 1965. Reciprocal patterns of genetic resistance to avian tumor viruses in two lines of chickens. Virology, 26: 664-672.

Vogt, P. K., and R. Ishizaki. 1966. Patterns of viral interference in the avian leukosis and sarcoma complex. Virology, 30: 368-374.

Witte, O. N., I. L. Weissman, and H. S. Kaplan. 1973. Structural characteristics of some murine RNA tumor viruses studied by lactoperoxidase iodination. Proc. Nat. Acad. Sci. U.S., 70: 36-40.

Witter, R., H. Frank, V. Moennig, G. Hunsmann, J. Lange, and W. Schäfer. 1973a. Properties of some mouse leukemia viruses. IV. Hemagglutination assay and characterization of hemagglutinating surface components. Virology, 54: 330-345.

Witter, R., G. Hunsmann, J. Lange, and W. Schäfer. 1973b. Properties of mouse leukemia viruses. V. Hemagglutination-inhibition and indirect hemagglutination tests. Virology, 54: 346-358.

Temperature-Sensitive Mutants of Avian Sarcoma Viruses

ROBERT R. FRIIS*
Department of Microbiology
University of Southern California Medical School
2025 Zonal Avenue
Los Angeles, California 90033

INTRODUCTION

THREE DIFFERENT categories of temperature-sensitive mutant avian sarcoma viruses may be distinguished on biological grounds: the replication mutants, which are defective for the production of infectious progeny virus at the nonpermissive temperature; the transformation mutants, which fail under such conditions to transform the host cell; and the coordinate function mutants, which are restricted at the nonpermissive temperature both for virus replication and host cell transformation. A number of the mutants have been further classified using biochemical and genetic techniques. These studies have shown that a less artificial assignment of mutants to categories is achieved if the organization is imposed on the principle of "early" and "late" viral functions.

Although the specific functional lesion has not been recognized for most mutants, simply because there is no known assay for most viral functions, inferences from the influences observed upon measurable functions make possible speculation about the mechanisms of replication and the patterns of regulation in the synthesis of viral progeny.

* Present address: Robert Koch-Institut des Bundesgesundheitsamtes, 1000 Berlin 65 West, Nordufer 20, Germany.

The Bryan high titer strain of Rous sarcoma virus (BH RSV) has provided an excellent precedent for the use of mutants in studies of avian RNA tumor viruses. This naturally defective virus fails to synthesize a functional envelope for progeny particles (Hanafusa et al., 1964) and has been reported to lack the major virion glycoprotein (Scheele and Hanafusa, 1971). The event that led to the emergence of this natural deletion mutant as the major avian sarcoma virus genotype among a heterogeneous population of avian leukosis viruses is unknown. In historical perspective it is clear that this mutant has played a central role in answering questions about the interactions of tumor viruses, such as the nature of phenotypic mixing among RNA tumor viruses (Vogt, 1967, 1968) and the phenomenon of expression of endogenous viral genetic information in normal chick embryo cells (Weiss, 1969; H. Hanafusa et al., 1970; Vogt and Friis, 1971).

The potential of temperature-sensitive mutants for answering a range of questions about the biology of RNA tumor viruses is much greater because such mutants may be obtained for each viral function, and since these mutants are conditional in their expression, clone-purified stocks may be readily obtained simply by using the permissive temperature (35 C). The influence of the specific lesion may be conveniently examined after performing an infection or shifting pre-infected cells to the nonpermissive temperature (41 C).

A substantial number of temperature-sensitive mutants already have been described. The majority may be briefly described as transformation-defective mutants (Martin, 1970; Bader and Brown, 1971; Kawai and Hanafusa, 1971; Biquard and Vigier, 1972; Wyke, 1973b). Mutants for which the replication of infectious progeny was restricted coordinately with transformation also have been described (Toyoshima and Vogt, 1969; Friis et al., 1971; Linial and Mason, 1973; and Wyke and Linial, 1973). The existence of a mutant which is defective only for replication of virus progeny has also been reported (Friis and Hunter, 1973). Studies dealing with the interrelationships of these mutants already have begun (Wyke, 1973b) and may be expected to yield a catalog of distinct physiologic and genetic groups. This paper will summarize the data from several laboratories, using a variety of techniques, which had as their common objective the identification of individual defective functions. This data indicated the existence of nine different types of temperature-sensitive mutants.

THE PROBLEM OF HOST GENETIC BACKGROUND

Phenotypic mixing of viral envelope proteins (Vogt, 1967) represents a kind of complementation event known to occur between different avian RNA tumor viruses infecting the same cell. A more direct kind of genetic interaction resulting in a reassortment of parental genetic markers in the progeny genome also has been described (Vogt, 1971; Kawai and Hanafusa, 1972). For this reason, studies of mutant RNA tumor viruses must be performed in a genetically homogeneous system, employing multiply cloned virus stocks and host cells which are free of expressed latent or endogenous viral genetic information. The problem of obtaining such a host cell is the central difficulty and theoretical objection to studies with these mutants.

Detection of the viral group-specific (*gs*) structural antigens and even whole virus particles in normal chick embryo tissue and tissue cultures (Dougherty et al., 1967) led to studies which demonstrated that expression of these markers for latent virus infection was inherited in chickens as a dominant, autosomal allele (Payne and Chubb, 1968). Subsequently, it was demonstrated that the production of an infectious, but nontransforming and probably nononcogenic, avian C-type virus occurred rarely as a spontaneous event (Vogt and Friis, 1971) and could be induced readily in normal chick embryo cells with physical and chemical carcinogens (Weiss et al., 1971). These carcinogen-induced viruses seem to be essentially identical to Rous associated virus 60 (RAV-60), a new virus detected (T. Hanafusa et al., 1970) in chick embryo cells after superinfection with avian sarcoma or leukosis viruses. However, although RAV-60 production could be observed only in chick embryo cells in which expression of latent viral functions could be detected beforehand, the induction of such viruses with carcinogens was possible even with chick embryo cells in which no detectable viral function could be observed prior to treatment. Since these viruses seem to be physically and biologically identical, it seems clear that essentially all sources of chick embryo cells contain a latent or endogenous C-type virus and that the cellular DNA possesses much of the genetic information of the avian sarcoma and leukosis viruses as measured by molecular hybridization (Varmus et al., 1972; Neiman, 1973). The degree of expression of such genetic information, and hence the availability of gene products and genetic material for complementation and recombination, respectively, is under regulation by a separate host locus.

The initial attempt to avoid this problem of the viral genetic background present in the chick embryo cells was to use Japanese quail cells, in which no detectable endogenous virus could be induced and in which only a small fraction of the avian sarcoma or leukosis virus genome could be detected by molecular hybridization (Varmus et al., 1972; Neiman, 1973). This approach failed because avian tumor viruses in general replicate very inefficiently in Japanese quail cells (Friis, 1972). Similar attempts with the duck host system, which also is free of detectable related endogenous viruses, were only partly successful, again because of the difficulty of obtaining efficient virus replication.

The only remaining solution to the problem of viral genetic background was adopted, although tentatively and with reservations. This approach was to select a population of chickens of which the progeny are, so far as can be determined, free of the expression of viral functions. Through the generous cooperation of R. Raymond, Heisdorf and Nelson Farms, Redmond, Washington, and E. Vielitz, Lohmann Tierzucht, Cuxhaven, Germany, such selected flocks have been obtained and extensively tested. Complement fixation tests were used to measure the viral *gs* antigens, and the chick helper factor test (T. Hanafusa et al., 1970) was employed to determine if the cells were competent to act as helpers for the defective BH RSV. Such embryos yield cells in tissue culture which have been maintained for as many as 12 passages without showing detectable expression of viral functions.

Chick embryo cells from such well-characterized sources have been used for these studies in the hope of reducing the possible effects of viral genetic background. It must be remembered, however, that our measures for expression of viral functions are limited to the detection of only a few viral structural proteins, and the expression of other viral functions may pass unnoticed. Hence, the nature of our host system may restrict investigation of mutants to studies of only those viral functions which cannot be complemented by the normal chick embryo cell.

THE ISOLATION OF TEMPERATURE-SENSITIVE MUTANTS

The technique of mutagenization with 5-azacytidine and isolation of temperature-sensitive mutants has been described by Toyoshima and Vogt (1969). For the present study mutagenized stocks of clone-purified Prague strains of Rous sarcoma virus (RSV), subgroup A (PR RSV-A) and subgroup C (PR RSV-C), and avian sarcoma virus B77, subgroup C, were plated at high dilution in a focus assay. Individual clones were isolated by aspiration of single foci, and each clone was tested for transformation of host cells and replication of progeny virus at both permissive and nonpermissive temperatures. At a frequency of approximately one raw mutant per hundred clonal isolates, temperature-sensitive mutants were obtained. Many of these proved to be leaky, and since in our laboratory an arbitrary convention has been established to the effect that useful mutants are defined as those in which transformation, replication, or both are suppressed of the order of 1,000-fold at the nonpermissive temperature, many raw mutants have been set aside without further characterization. It is possible that our convention excludes mutants in certain functions from study, but for operational reasons some limit of acceptable leakiness must be defined. In addition to leakiness, reversion to the wild type may occur in mutant stocks; hence, for reliable stocks, virus cloning must be repeated at each step, and individual stock clones must be tested separately for the temperature sensitivity and level of leakiness before use in experiments.

FUNCTIONAL CLASSIFICATION OF TEMPERATURE-SENSITIVE MUTANTS

The initial and obvious markers for study of mutants with RNA tumor viruses are the transformation of the host cell, which can be produced with sarcoma viruses, and the replication of progeny viruses. Somewhere along the path at the beginning of mutant characterization studies, someone coined the phrase "coordinate mutants" to describe those mutants which failed in both basic biological functions, and it was easy to refer to the more restricted defectives as "transformation mutants" or "replication mutants."

Somewhat more sophisticated tests also can be applied within the framework of biological experiments. The temperature-shift experiment is such a test, with very simple manipulations, which yields important results. Cells which have been infected with mutants may be maintained initially at either the permissive temperature or the nonpermissive temperature. If the permissive temperature (35 C) is chosen, then the cultures express phenotypically wild-type properties of infection. If then, at some later time, the temperature is shifted to the nonpermissive temperature (41 C), a very interesting question can be answered in observing whether or not the mutants exhibit a defective function. If not, then one may assume that the temperature-sensitive function is one which must act transiently; once the infection has progressed beyond this block, it is irreversibly established regardless of the incubation temperature. For example, the provirus hypothesis of Temin (1964), which has been strengthened theoretically by the finding that a reverse transcriptase or RNA-dependent DNA polymerase is present in RNA tumor viruses (Baltimore, 1970; Temin and Mizutani, 1970), would predict such a requirement for a transient function. The reverse transcriptase must play such a role early in infection by producing a DNA provirus from the entering viral RNA genome. After this function has occured, the provirus is present in the nucleus of the cell, and even a temperature-sensitive reverse transcriptase will not cripple the infection if the shift to the nonpermissive temperature is applied after the provirus DNA is complete.

The temperature-shift procedure also can be applied in the converse experiment. Cells can be infected initially with mutants at the nonpermissive temperature and later subjected to a shift to the permissive temperature. In this case, one would expect that a mutant with an early transient-function defect would be irreversibly destroyed, and infection could not progress further. On the other hand, most late-function mutants, in which the early transient functions have been successfully completed at the nonpermissive temperature, simply produce proteins at both temperatures. If temperature sensitive, the mutants are nonfunctional so long as the cells are incubated at the nonpermissive temperature, but are functional as soon as synthesis can be effected at the permissive temperature. In this way, the time necessary for a shift from nonpermissive to permissive temperatures to take effect (producing a change to phenotypically wild-type expression of viral functions) can give a rough idea of whether the defect occurs just before synthesis of mature virus or at an earlier stage, where proteins act in an enzymatic or regulatory role.

Another biological procedure is the complementation test. This procedure involves establishing a mixed infection of two different viruses—mutants or wild types—in the same cell. It is known that some viral functions can be shared; that is, phenotypically mixed virus particles can be produced (Vogt, 1967), whereas others probably cannot be. For example, the reverse transcriptase is such a function which apparently can act only upon the RNA genome with which it entered the cell (unpub. obs.). With this test, mutants may be grouped functionally according to whether or not they can assist each other in mixed infection. This procedure offers many technical problems and has not been applied completely except to the transformation mutants studied by Wyke (1973a).

Biochemical and immunological tools also have been applied to the characterization of mutants. Mutant virus preparations may be tested *in vitro* for temperature-sensitive reverse transcriptase activity (Linial and Mason, 1973). Molecular hybridization has been applied to determine if temperature-sensitive mutant-infected cells produce new progeny viral RNA at the nonpermissive temperature (pers. comm., J. M. Bishop). The presence of viral group-specific antigens (*gs* antigens) in cells at the nonpermissive temperature also has been the subject of radioimmuno-precipitation studies (Halpern et al., 1974). Other more sophisticated biochemical procedures will certainly be used to answer questions about each step of virus replication. We hope that the use of these techniques with mutants will enable us to recognize viral functions which have intractable properties in analysis of wild-type viruses.

Characteristics for nine different kinds of mutants are presented. These mutants, based on the approaches to classification described above, have been organized as "early," "late transformation," and "late replication" mutants. Information dealing with these mutants is very limited, or not fully confirmed. Therefore, this identification of different kinds of mutants is tentative and speculative. We believe this organization to be useful, however, because it suggests many biochemical and genetic experiments.

Early Mutants

The provirus hypothesis of Temin (1964) still best explains the complex chain of events that leads to incorporation of the RNA tumor virus genetic information into the chromosomal DNA of the host cell. Figure 1, in conjunction with Table 1, correlates our data from the various mutants with the recognized processes in the pathway of virus replication and virus-induced host cell transformation. The first step (code no. 1) designates mutants defective in the function required for the synthesis of the DNA provirus. These may be simply visualized as mutants with a defective reverse transcriptase.

Figure 1.   A diagram in which the various types of specific data mentioned in the text are correlated, resulting in a speculative sequence of viral functional events. Some of these proposed steps are recognized and accepted on the basis of known biochemical data; others may be proposed only on the basis of mutant behavior and characteristics. A code number located next to each small cross indicates the proposed functional block associated with the various mutants tabulated in Table 1.

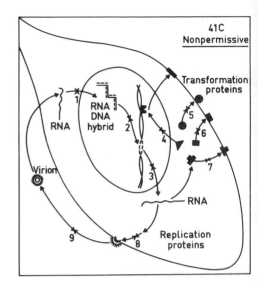

Ts 335 and *ts* 337 are mutants of this type (Linial and Mason, 1973; W. S. Mason, pers. comm.). *In vitro* assays have shown conclusively that reverse transcriptase activity is temperature sensitive. Furthermore, ribonuclease H (RNase H), the RNA:DNA hybrid-specific nuclease (Molling et al., 1971), is apparently borne at a second enzymatic site on the same enzyme complex and is also detectably temperature sensitive (D. Baltimore, pers. comm.). The known biological and biochemical characteristics of infection with these mutants (Table 1) are consistent with an early transient function defect. No viral functions whatever can be detected in cells which are infected at the nonpermissive temperature, whether or not the cells are subsequently shifted to the permissive temperature. Furthermore, once the infection has been established at the permissive temperature, effective replication and transformation of the host cells are not abolished by a shift to the nonpermissive temperature. As might be predicted, the virions of these mutants are somewhat temperature sensitive, and inactivation of infectivity by incubation at 41 C occurs about twice as rapidly with the mutant as with the wild type.

The function prohibited by the second step (code no. 2) has no counterpart in the known biochemical events of early infection. The initial recognition of an "early" mutant on the basis of its response in a temperature-shift experiment was described by Friis and coworkers (1971) for *ts* 336 (originally *ts* 149). Subsequently it has

Table 1. Properties of infection at the nonpermissive temperature

Code no.	Mutants	Isolated by	Provirus DNA	Provirus integration	RNA transcription	Viral envelope antigen synthesis	Group-specific antigen synthesis	Particle production	Productive infection	Transformation
1	335	Wyke	−	−	−	−	−	−	−	−
	337	Mason	−	−	−	−	−	−	−	−
2	336	Toyo-shima	+	−	−	−	−	−	−	−
3	338	Wyke	+	+	−	−	−	−	−	−
	343	Linial	+	+	−	−	−	−	−	−
4	25	Wyke	+	+	+	+	+	+	+	−
	33	Wyke	+	+	+	+	+	+	+	−
5	23	Wyke	+	+	+	+	+	+	+	−
6	24	Wyke	+	+	+	+	+	+	+	−
7	29	Wyke	+	+	+	+	+	+	+	−
8	334	Toyo-shima	+	+	+	−	+	−	−	−
9	672	Friis	+	+	+	+	+	+	−	+

been shown that although *ts* 336 exhibits the same shift properties as *ts* 335 and *ts* 337, namely those characteristic of a mutant defective in an early transient, rapidly labile function, *ts* 336 has a reverse transcriptase which is no more temperature sensitive in *in vitro* assays than is the wild type. Thus, one must speculate about a separate essential early function. Additional data obtained from phenotypic mixing experiments have shown that the defective function in *ts* 336 must be brought into the cell with the infecting virion, since it can be complemented in stocks prepared with avian leukosis helper viruses. As shown in Table 1, except for the apparently viable reverse transcriptase, *ts* 336 is identical to code no. 1 mutants in that it fails to display any viral functions upon infection at the nonpermissive temperature. The destruction is irreversible since a subsequent shift to the permissive temperature fails to restore infection.

The third step (code no. 3) indicates the function responsible for regulating or inducing transcription of the integrated viral genetic information. Since it has been arbitrarily agreed that the designation "early" mutants should apply only to those showing an irreversible defect caused by loss of an early transient function, the function denoted by code no. 3 must be discussed as a "late" defect.

Late Coordinate Mutants—*ts* 338 and *ts* 343

The mutants designated by code no. 3 have caused a great deal of confusion because they are characterized by a reversible defect that affects both replication and transformation (Wyke and Linial, 1973). To further confuse the issues, *ts* 338 must be at least a double mutant with a second lesion influencing exclusively the late transformation events (D. Blair, pers. comm.). These mutants, furthermore, are amenable to complementation; i.e., in mixed infection with avian leukosis helper viruses, the defective function can be complemented. Biochemical studies have presented us with a comprehensible explanation (Fig. 1). Molecular hybridization experiments conducted by J. M. Bishop (pers. comm.) show that at the nonpermissive temperature *ts* 338 and *ts* 343 fail to make progeny viral RNA transcripts. All of the data concerning these mutants can best be explained by saying that a lesion similar to the one shown by code no. 3 prevents the normal transcription of viral RNA from the integrated proviral DNA. Whether this defective function is a regulatory one or an enzymatic one is unknown.

Late Transformation Mutants

The transformation mutants are those which are able to replicate their progeny, but are unable to transform the host cell at the nonpermissive temperature. A great number have been isolated by Wyke (1973a) using a selective technique, and have been arranged into four complementation groups on the basis of the only complete complementation studies yet performed in this system (Wyke, 1973a). In our diagram four code numbers (4, 5, 6, and 7) have been devoted to Wyke's complementation groups. Three refer to sites of action at the membrane. This reference is purely diagrammatic and does not suggest any localization. In fact, absolutely nothing is known about the nature of the transformation functions indicated except that, on the basis of complementation tests, they are distinct. Code no. 4, the exception, indicates a site of action at the host cell chromosome.

Preliminary observations indicate that for the successful restoration of function, i.e., host cell phenotypic transformation, these mutants require new host RNA synthesis as well as new protein synthesis. These data were obtained with actinomycin D inhibition studies performed under well-controlled conditions, but require confirmation with other techniques. If these data are correct, however, they suggest that at least one of the transformation-mutant complementation groups is defective in a function which is presumed to act in regulating some host cell genetic information. It is easy to visualize viral-induced transformation taking place by means of such a mechanism.

A variety of transformation markers are available for analysis. In addition to the property of producing foci under agar overlay, avian sarcoma virus-infected cells also characteristically produce colonies in soft agar suspension culture. Furthermore, transformed cells exhibit unique antigens associated with a specific viral etiology (Kurth and Bauer, 1973). Hatanaka and Hanafusa (1970) have described significant alterations in the rate of uptake of certain sugars after transformation, especially the increased rate of uptake of the nonmetabolized sugar 2-deoxyglucose. Many of the characteristics of transformed cells have been examined with mutant-infected cells at both temperatures. It has been found, for example, that the ability to produce soft agar colonies is not necessarily temperature sensitive for mutants which have lost the ability to produce foci under agar overlay (Wyke and Linial, 1973). The expression of particular antigens specific for transformation of cells with avian sarcoma viruses may or may not be temperature sensitive, depending on the mutant examined (pers. comm., R. Kurth). Of the typical measures of transformation, only the increased rate of 2-deoxyglucose uptake has been shown to correlate perfectly with the transformed state of the cell, as indicated by the stringent focus test. These results indicate that transformation is a continuum of interacting alterations in cell behavior and biochemistry, each being determined by one or more viral functions which either act at a site in the cell directly or influence the cell indirectly by action on the genetic material to alter and transform the cell.

The study of transforming functions is certainly the most interesting area of this research, although the most difficult, and is the only such research absolutely relevant to the study of cancer. It is hoped that these mutants may be useful in this field. Great promise is offered by the approach of Graf and Friis (1973), which is to use avian sarcoma virus mutants to transform mammalian cells which can then be maintained, cloned, and studied with respect to the more universal properties of transformation.

Late Replication Mutants

Code nos. 8 and 9 (Table 1) refer to mutants which are blocked in the replication of infectious progeny, although other viral functions such as transformation are not impaired. Various structural antigens may be recognized in the cells. These are termed "late" replication mutants. The first late mutant defined, ts 334 (originally ts 75 Friis et al., 1971), proved to be atypical in that both transformation and replication were affected, although from the rapid restoration of virus production after temperature shift to the permissive temperature, it was apparent from the beginning that the defect must be a "late" function. This anomaly, the temperature sensitivity of transformation, was recently explained by Owada and Toyoshima (1973) when they demonstrated that ts 334 has a second late-transformation mutant lesion. This result has been confirmed by showing that reversion of the transformation-defective lesion occurs independently of the late replication-defective function.

Additional studies with ts 334 have shown that while few physical particles are made by infected cells at the nonpermissive temperature, group-specific antigens are made and processed normally (Katz and Vogt, 1971). Ts 334 fails, however, to synthesize viral envelope antigen, according to results with immunofluorescent procedures (Halpern et al., 1974). Also, it does not generate interfering activity in infected cells at the nonpermissive temperature, which would be expected if viral envelope antigen synthesis were taking place. Hence, the data available suggest that *ts* 334 is defective in a step which leads to the production of viral envelope antigen. The viral envelope antigen is, however, a glycoprotein, so synthesis may involve the interaction of several cistrons of viral genetic information. Comparison studies have been made between *ts* 334 and BH RSV, which is known to be defective with respect to the synthesis of a functional viral envelope (Hanafusa et al., 1964; Scheele and Hanafusa, 1971). Results of such studies show that these two defective viruses must have lesions in different functions since they are able to complement each other in mixed infections.

Another "late" replication mutant, *ts* 672, is designated by code no. 9. This mutant completes, in a sense, the cycle of presently recognized viral functions. *Ts* 672 has been shown to induce host cell transformation and to synthesize noninfectious virus physical particles at the nonpermissive temperature (Friis and Hunter, 1973). Further investigation of the noninfectious physical particles produced at 41 C demonstrates they lack reverse transcriptase activity and, therefore, are noninfectious because no DNA provirus can be synthesized. Since the infectious particles made at the permissive temperature exhibit no particular temperature sensitivity in early infection and the reverse transcriptase from these infectious viruses is not temperature sensitive in *in vitro* tests, it must be concluded that *ts* 672 has a lesion which is temperature sensitive only when the reverse transcriptase is being synthesized or assembled. This lesion occurs prior to the release of the noninfectious progeny.

Significance

The study of mutants, especially of a chicken virus, is obviously an academic pursuit. We believe there will be results of general significance, however, and can point now to the early and coordinate functions, code nos. 2 and 3, for which no biochemical evidence exists. In the area of cancer research, general significance may be expected from the analysis of functions which act on the host at the genetic level versus those which act on a specific cellular site.

Acknowledgments: This study was supported by research grant number CA 13213 and by contract number NCI 72-2032 from the National Cancer Institute. The information summarized here was obtained through the collaborative efforts of a number of people, in particular H. Bauer, J. M. Bishop, M. S. Halpern, R. Kurth, W. S. Mason, K. Mölling, and J. A. Wyke. I would like to thank them for their practical help and useful discussions, as well as for permission to mention certain incomplete or preliminary data.

Literature Cited

Bader, J. P., and N. R. Brown. 1971. Induction of mutations in an RNA tumor virus by an analog of a DNA precursor. Nature New Biol., *234:* 11-12.

Baltimore, D. 1970. RNA-dependent DNA polymerase in virions of RNA tumor viruses. Nature (London), *226:* 1209-1211.

Biquard, J., and P. Vigier. 1970. Isolement et étude d'un mutant conditionnel du virus de Rous à capacité transformante thermosensible. Comptes Rendus Acad. Sci. ser. D., *271:* 2430-2433.

Dougherty, R. M., H. S. DiStefano, and F. K. Roth. 1967. Virus particles and viral antigens in chicken tissues free of infectious avian leukosis virus. Proc. Nat. Acad. Sci. U.S., *58:* 808-817.

Friis, R. R. 1972. Abortive infection of Japanese quail cells with avian sarcoma viruses. Virology, *50:* 701-712.

Friis, R. R., and E. Hunter. 1973. Temperature sensitive mutant of Rous sarcoma virus that is defective for replication. Virology, *53:* 479-483.

Friis, R. R., K. Toyoshima, and P. K. Vogt. 1971. Conditional lethal mutants of avian sarcoma viruses. I. Physiology of *ts* 75 and *ts* 149. Virology, *43:* 375-389.

Graf, T., and R. R. Friis. 1973. Differential expression of transformation in rat and chicken cells infected with avian sarcoma virus temperature sensitive mutant. Virology, *56:* 369-374.

Halpern, M. S., E. Hunter, M. C. Alevy, R. R. Friis, and P. K. Vogt. 1974. Viral-specific protein in cells infected with two temperature sensitive mutants of avian sarcoma viruses. In preparation.

Hanafusa, H., T. Hanafusa, and H. Rubin. 1964. Analysis of the defectiveness of Rous sarcoma virus. II. Specification of RSV antigenicity by helper virus. Proc. Nat. Acad. Sci. U.S., *51:* 41-48.

Hanafusa, H., T. Miyamoto, and T. Hanafusa. 1970. A cell-associated factor essential for formation of an infectious form of Rous sarcoma virus. Proc. Nat. Acad. Sci. U.S., *66:* 314-321.

Hanafusa, T., H. Hanafusa, and T. Miyamoto. 1970. Recovery of a new virus from apparently normal chick cells by infection with avian tumor viruses. Proc. Nat. Acad. Sci. U.S., *67:* 1797-1803.

Hatanaka, M., and H. Hanafusa. 1970. Analysis of a functional change in membrane in the process of cell transformation by Rous sarcoma virus: Alteration in the characteristics of sugar transport. Virology, *41:* 647-652.

Katz, E., and P. K. Vogt. 1971. Conditional lethal mutants of avian sarcoma viruses. II. Analysis of the temperature sensitive lesion in *ts* 75. Virology *46:* 745-753.

Kawai, S., and H. Hanafusa. 1971. The effects of reciprocal changes in temperature on the transformed state of cells infected with a Rous sarcoma virus mutant. Virology, *46:* 470-479.

Kawai, S., and H. Hanafusa. 1972. Genetic recombination with avian tumor viruses. Virology, *49:* 37-44.

Kurth, R., and H. Bauer. 1973. Avian oncornavirus-induced tumor antigens of embryonic and unknown origin. Virology, *56:* 496-504.

Linial, M., and W. S. Mason. 1973. Characterization of two conditional early mutants of Rous sarcoma virus. Virology, *53:* 258-273.

Martin, G. S. 1970. Rous sarcoma virus: A function required for maintenance of the transformed state. Nature (London), *227:* 1021-1022.

Mölling, K., D. P. Bolognesi, H. Bauer, W. Büsen, H. W. Plassmann, and P. Hausen. 1971. Association of viral reverse transcriptase with an enzyme degrading the RNA moiety of RNA-DNA hybrids. Nature New Biol., *234:* 240-243.

Neiman, P. 1973. Measurement of endogenous leukosis virus nucleotide sequences in the DNA of normal avian embryos by RNA-DNA hybridization. Virology, *53:* 196-204.

Owada, M., and K. Toyoshima. 1973. Analysis on the reproducing and cell-transforming capacities of a temperature sensitive mutant (*ts* 334) of avian sarcoma virus B77. Virology, *54:* 170-178.

Payne, L. N., and R. C. Chubb. 1968. Studies on the nature and genetic control of an antigen in normal chick embryos which reacts in the COFAL test. J. Gen. Virol., *3:* 379-391.

Scheele, C., and H. Hanafusa. 1971. Proteins of helper-dependent RSV. Virology, *45:* 401-410.

Temin, H. M. 1964. Nature of the provirus of Rous sarcoma. Nat. Cancer Inst. Mono., *17:* 557-570.

Temin, H. M., and S. Mizutani. 1970. RNA-dependent DNA polymerase in virions of Rous sarcoma virus. Nature (London), *226:* 1211-1213.

Toyoshima, K., and P. K. Vogt. 1969. Temperature sensitive mutants of avian sarcoma virus. Virology, *39:* 930-931.

Varmus, H. E., R. A. Weiss, R. R. Friis, W. Levinson, and J. M. Bishop. 1972. Detection of avian tumor virus-specific nucleotide sequences in avian cell DNAs. Proc. Nat. Acad. Sci. U.S., *69:* 20-24.

Vogt, P. K. 1967. Phenotypic mixing in the avian tumor virus group. Virology, *32:* 708-717.

Vogt, P. K. 1968. Cooperative and antagonistic interactions among RNA tumor viruses. Nat. Cancer Inst. Mono., *29:* 421-426.

Vogt, P. K. 1971. Genetically stable reassortment of markers during mixed infection with avian tumor viruses. Virology, *46:* 947-952.

Vogt, P. K., and R. R. Friis. 1971. An avian leukosis virus related to RSV(0): Properties and evidence for helper activity. Virology, *43:* 223-234.

Weiss, R. A. 1969. Interference and neutralization studies with Bryan strain Rous sarcoma virus synthesized in the absence of helper virus. J. Gen. Virol., *5:* 529-539.

Weiss, R. A., R. R. Friis, E. Katz, and P. K. Vogt. 1971. Induction of avian tumor viruses in normal cells by physical and chemical carcinogens. Virology, *46*: 920-938.

Wyke, J. A. 1973a. The selective isolation of temperature sensitive mutants of Rous sarcoma virus. Virology, *52*: 587-590.

Wyke, J. A. 1973b. Complementation of transforming functions by temperature sensitive mutants of avian sarcoma virus. Virology, *54*: 28-36.

Wyke, J. A., and M. Linial. 1973. Temperature sensitive avian sarcoma viruses: A physiological comparison of twenty mutants. Virology, *53*: 152-161.

The Avian Myeloblastosis Virus RNA-Dependent DNA Polymerase

J. Leis, J. Hurwitz, A. L. Schincariol,
M. Stone, and W. K. Joklik*
Duke University Medical Center
Department of Microbiology and Immunology
Durham, North Carolina 27706

INTRODUCTION

HIGHLY PURIFIED preparations of avian myeloblastosis virus DNA polymerase catalyze repairlike reactions on RNA, DNA, or RNA-DNA hybrids. Deoxynucleotide incorporation occurs specifically from 3′ OH ends of primer strands attached to template strands. The newly synthesized DNA is small (6-7S) when analyzed by alkaline sucrose gradients. A protein, isolated from AMV, stimulated DNA synthesis but had no effect on the size of the DNA formed.

Purified preparations of RNA-dependent DNA polymerase isolated from avian myeloblastosis virus also contain RNase H activity. Removal of the DNA polymer at any time during the reaction stops the degradation of RNA. The nuclease has been characterized as a processive exonuclease which requires poly(A) chains with ends for activity. Attack on poly(A) modified at 5′ or 3′ ends occurs, indicating that the enzyme acts in both the 5′ to 3′ and 3′ to 5′ directions. RNase H does not yield detectable amounts of acid-soluble [^{32}P] from 60S viral RNA labeled with [^{32}P] during DNA synthesis with purified reverse transcriptase. The significance of these observations

* At the time this paper was presented, J. Leis and J. Hurwitz were affiliated with Albert Einstein College of Medicine, Department of Developmental Biology and Cancer, 1300 Morris Park Avenue, Bronx, New York 10461.

and the possible role that RNase H plays in tumor virus RNA replication are discussed.

RNA tumor viruses appear to replicate via a DNA intermediate. This conclusion is supported by the observation that virus infection is blocked by inhibitors of DNA synthesis (Bader, 1964; Temin, 1964; Vigier and Golde, 1964) and by the presence of an enzyme capable of transcribing viral RNA into DNA, RNA-dependent DNA polymerase, in virions (Baltimore, 1970; Temin and Mizutani, 1970). Purified RNA-dependent DNA polymerase catalyzes repairlike DNA synthesis with RNA, DNA, and RNA-DNA hybrids. The enzyme requires primer strands containing 3′ OH termini which serve as initiation sites attached to template strands which direct DNA synthesis (Duesberg et al., 1971; Smoler et al., 1971; Verma et al., 1971; Hurwitz and Leis, 1972; Leis and Hurwitz, 1972; Taylor et al., 1972). The product of the reaction with AMV RNA is an RNA-DNA covalent hybrid (Leis and Hurwitz, 1972; Verma et al., 1972), and the newly synthesized DNA is small (5-7S as shown by alkaline sucrose gradient analysis).

Recently, Mölling and co-workers (1971) reported that ribonuclease H (RNase H), an enzyme which specifically degrades polyribonucleotides in RNA-DNA hybrids, was not separated from avian myeloblastosis virus (AMV) polymerase on purification. These authors proposed that RNase H activity, in conjunction with the AMV polymerase, played an important role in the generation of free DNA from RNA-DNA transcript products. The presence of RNase H activity in preparations of purified RNA-dependent DNA polymerase has been confirmed in several laboratories (Mölling et al., 1971; Baltimore and Smoler, 1972; Grandgenett et al., 1972; Keller and Crouch, 1972; Leis et al., 1973; Watson et al., 1973). However, the function of RNase H in transcription of viral RNA is not clear.

An additional protein, referred to as stimulatory protein (Leis and Hurwitz, 1972b), has also been isolated from AMV. This protein is associated with reverse transcriptase during purification but can be separated from the polymerase by repeated phosphocellulose chromatography. As previously reported (Leis and Hurwitz, 1972b) stimulatory protein alters some properties of reverse transcriptase. The present paper presents evidence that the AMV RNase H acts as a processive exonuclease, reports additional studies on stimulatory protein, and discusses the possible role of these activities in the transcription of RNA of oncornavirus.

RNase H activity associated with AMV polymerase

AMV polymerase, purified as previously described (Leis and Hurwitz, 1972b), has detectable RNase H activity, as measured by acid-solubilization of [³H]poly(A) in the presence of poly(dT). In addition, AMV polymerase preparations isolated after chromatography on IRC-50 or DNA-agarose contain RNase H activity. Although RNase H is closely associated with polymerase activity, as measured by DNA synthesis primed by AMV 60S RNA or d(AT) copolymer, the two activities are not always coincidental. The ratio of DNA synthesis to poly(A) degradation has varied as much as 2 to 3 fold across the enzyme peak eluted from phosphocellulose (Leis et al., 1973).

Comparison of properties of RNase H and DNA polymerase

AMV polymerase and RNase H, in general, exhibit identical requirements for metal, sulfhydryl reagents, and pH. Requirements for DNA polymerase were as previously described (Hurwitz and Leis, 1972; Leis and Hurwitz, 1972a). Optimal RNase H activity was observed with 10 to 12 mM $MgCl_2$; at concentrations greater than 12 mM, activity decreased. Mn^{+2} ions can only partially replace Mg^{+2} ions for activity; in this case, optimal activity was observed with 0.2-0.3 mM Mn^{+2}. The degradation of [³H]poly(A) is dependent upon the presence of poly(dT) and there is no detectable breakdown of the DNA polymer during the course of the reaction. Both RNase H and polymerase activities are influenced by the presence of salt. RNase H activity was inhibited 50 percent by 0.13 M KCl while DNA synthesis, measured by d(AT) copolymer synthesis, was inhibited 50 percent by 0.08 M KCl. In contrast to the action of polymerase, RNase H activity does not depend on the presence of deoxynucleotides. RNase H activity measured in the presence of all four deoxynucleoside triphosphates or dTTP alone was hardly affected.

The rate of degradation of [³H]poly(A) (300-400 nucleotides in length) in the presence of poly(dT) was linear until approximately 60 percent of the poly(A) was rendered acid-soluble. The rate decreased at this point, though the reaction continued until more than 95 percent of the poly(A) was degraded. Under the standard assay conditions, the rate of RNase H action was proportional to added purified enzyme up to a 0.2 unit of polymerase.

Antibodies prepared by R. Nowinski of the University of Wisconsin against preparations of AMV reverse transcriptase, isolated as described by Kacian and co-workers (1971), were found to also neutralize RNase H activity of our enzyme preparations. The antibodies specifically neutralized AMV RNase H and had no effect on RNase H isolated from *Escherichia coli*. In addition, antibodies prepared against a DNA polymerase isolated from chick embryo cells affected neither transcriptase nor RNase H activities.

Although RNase H and DNA polymerase have similar requirements for activity, they can be distinguished by the differences in

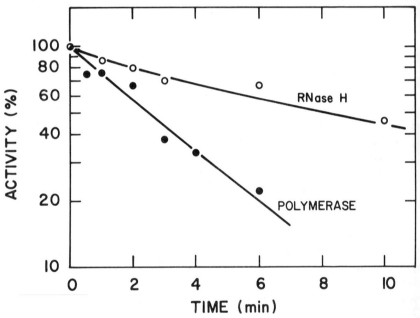

Figure 1.   Effect of heat on AMV RNase H and DNA polymerase activities. Purified AMV polymerase was incubated at 48 C and at times indicated aliquots (0.16 unit polymerase) were removed and placed on ice. Treated samples were assayed for either RNase H with [³H]poly(A) (32 cpm/pmole, 1.12 nmoles) and poly(dT) (1.0 nmole) or DNA synthesis measured by d(AT) copolymer synthesis with [³H]dTTP (257 cpm/pmole, 0.88 nmole), dATP (1 nmole), and d(AT) copolymer (1.95 nmoles) as described in Methods except that both assays contained 12 μg/ml bovine serum albumin and 5 mM KCl. One nmole of unlabeled TTP was added to the incubation for RNase H assay. Activity of untreated enzyme was taken as 100 percent. These values were: d(AT) copolymer synthesis, 157 pmoles; RNase H activity, 241 pmoles. DNA polymerase, ●——————●; RNase H, O————O.

their sensitivities to heat or N-ethylmaleimide (NEM). Polymerase activity is more sensitive to inactivation by heat than RNase H, in agreement with the results of Mölling and co-workers (1971); 50 percent of the polymerase activity was inactivated in 2.5 minutes at 48 C, while 50 percent of the more stable RNase H activity was inactivated after 9.5 minutes at 48 C (Fig. 1). Treatment of purified enzyme preparations with sulfhydryl-reacting reagents such as p-hydroxymercuribenzoate (pHMB) or NEM inactivated both enzyme activities. Incubation of purified polymerase (0.22 unit) and stimulatory protein (23 ng) with pHMB under assay conditions used for the data in Figure 2 resulted in 50 percent inhibition of RNase H activity with 0.3 to 0.4 mM pHMB; polymerase activity was inhibited 50 percent with 0.8 to 0.9 mM pHMB. At 2 mM pHMB both activities were completely blocked. In contrast to observations with pHMB, RNase H activity was relatively resistant to inactivation by NEM (Fig. 2). At concentrations of 3 mM NEM, AMV polymerase activity was completely inhibited while RNase H activity was still detected in the presence of 20 mM NEM. These observations suggest that RNase H and DNA polymerase activities occur at different active catalytic sites. This conclusion is consistent with the observations described above in which RNase H and DNA polymerase activities were not always coincidentally eluted from phosphocellulose columns. To date, however, we have not isolated polymerase fractions devoid of RNase H activity.

Effect of stimulatory protein on RNase H

An auxiliary protein fraction has been isolated from AMV which specifically stimulates the rate of DNA synthesis by purified reverse transcriptase primed with 60S AMV RNA preparations (Leis and Hurwitz, 1972b). The extent of this stimulation appears to depend on the nature of the primer RNA. A 6 to 8 fold stimulation occurred with RNA preparations that yield a large proportion of 20S RNA fragments upon denaturation. With more intact RNA preparations the stimulation of rate is only 2 to 3 fold. The stimulatory protein fraction also increased the rate of attack of AMV RNase H on [^{3}H]poly(A)·poly(dT) (Table 1). In the absence of polymerase, the stimulatory protein was free of detectable RNase H activity. As observed for DNA synthesis, the stimulatory protein specifically affected AMV RNase H and had no effect on RNase H purified from *E. coli*. Incubation of stimulatory protein with 20 mM NEM at 25 C

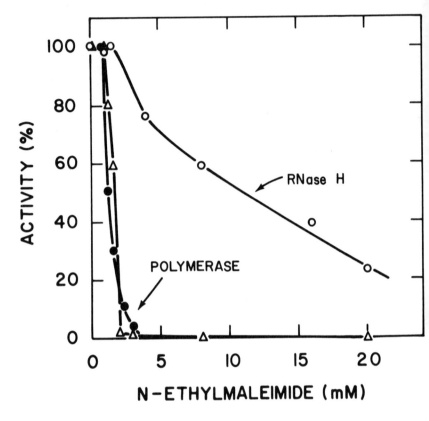

Figure 2.   Effect of NEM on AMV RNase H and DNA polymerase activities. Purified polymerase preparations (0.22 unit) and stimulatory protein (23 ng) were incubated with various concentrations of NEM under DNA polymerase and RNase H assay conditions except that dithioerythritol and albumin were omitted and incubations were carried out in 50 percent glycerol. RNase H was measured by amount of [³H]poly(A) (0.56 nmo!e, 32 cpm/pmole) rendered acid-soluble in the presence of poly(dT) (0.52 nmole) after 10 minutes of incubation at 38 C, while DNA synthesis was measured by incorporation of [³H]dTTP (1 nmole, 459 cpm/pmole) in response to d(AT) copolymer (1.98 nmo!es) after 10 minutes at 38 C or [³H]dCTP (1 nmole, 1,300 cpm/pmole) and dATP, dGTP, dTTP (each 5 nmoles) in response to AMV RNA (480 pmoles) after 15 minutes at 38 C into acid-insoluble material. Activity in the absence of NEM taken as 100 percent represented 107 pmoles [³H]poly(A) degraded, 13.1 pmoles dTMP incorporated with dAT copolymer as primer, and 0.67 pmole dCMP incorporated with AMV RNA. RNase H, O————O; DNA synthesis primed with AMV RNA, ●————●; DNA synthesis primed with d(AT) copolymer, △————△.

Table 1.   Influence of AMV stimulatory protein on degradation of
poly(A)·poly(dT)

Additions	[³H]poly(A) rendered acid-soluble
	pmoles/30 min.
AMV polymerase[1]	56
AMV stimulatory protein (23 ng)	2
AMV polymerase + AMV stimulatory protein (23 ng)	220
AMV polymerase + AMV stimulatory protein[2]	56
E. coli RNase H (43 ng)	41
E. coli RNase H + AMV stimulatory protein (23 ng)	29

[1] 0.22 units of AMV polymerase was used and assay was carried out as described in Methods.

[2] In this experiment, AMV stimulatory protein was treated with pronase as follows: Pronase (5 mg/ml) was self-digested for 2 hours at 45 C, then heated at 80 C for 2 minutes. Stimulatory protein (228 ng) was incubated for 27 hours at 38 C with 500 μg pronase and then assayed for stimulation of RNase H activity. Stimulatory protein without pronase was incubated 27 hours at 30 C as a control.

for 5 minutes, followed by removal of unreacted NEM with 0.26 M 2-mercaptoethanol, did not affect its stimulation of RNase activity.

The role that stimulatory protein plays during transcription of tumor virus RNA is unclear. The factor stimulates the rate of DNA synthesis and RNase H activity, enables the polymerase to initiate DNA synthesis from single-strand breaks in duplex DNA, and appears to increase the release of DNA with small pieces of RNA covalently linked from the 60S RNA complex *in vitro* (Leis and Hurwitz, 1972b). It does not, however, greatly affect the size range of 6 to 7S DNA synthesized *in vitro* with "intact" 60S RNA as analyzed on alkaline sucrose gradients (Fig. 3) but rather increases the amount of smaller pieces of DNA synthesized. This result indicates that the factor increases the number of available DNA synthesis initiation sites and suggests that stimulatory protein is probably not an unwinding protein as described by Alberts (1967). The latter proteins appear to interact with single-stranded DNAs and render them resistant to the action of *Neurospora* nuclease. The stimulatory protein does not protect single-stranded RNAs from attack by this nuclease.

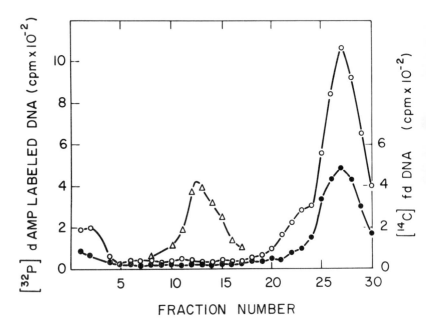

Figure 3.   Influence of stimulatory protein on the size of DNA products. Puri-fied AMV polymerase (0.65 unit) was incubated in a 0.2 ml reaction mixture with or without stimulatory protein (78.4 ng) containing AMV RNA (1.94 nmoles), [α-³²ᵖ] dATP (4.1 nmoles, 5.450 cpm/pmole), and dGTP, dCTP, dTTP (each 20 nmoles) as described in Methods. After 60 minutes at 38 C, the reaction was stopped by the addition of 20 μmoles EDTA. Reaction mixture lacking stimulatory protein incorporated 12,600 cpm into acid-insoluble mate-rial while reaction mixtures with polymerase and stimulatory protein contained 51,080 cpm. Extraction and sucrose gradient procedures are given in Methods. In this figure, DNA prepared without stimulatory protein is indicated by the symbols, ●————●; products synthesized in the presence of stimulatory pro-tein are represented by the symbols, O————O; [¹⁴C] fd DNA, △————△.

Studies with Rauscher polymerase

Previous studies from this laboratory (Hurwitz and Leis, 1972; Leis and Hurwitz, 1972a) and others (Scolnick et al., 1970; Spiegel-man et al., 1970) have reported similarities between DNA poly-merase activity isolated from Rauscher leukemia virions (RLV) and that isolated from AMV. This similarity is striking when synthetic polynucleotides such as poly(A)·poly(dT) (Table 2) or DNA (properly altered) is used as primer-template. However, to date, we have had no success in isolating Rauscher polymerase preparations

Table 2.   Activities of viral polymerases

Expt.[1]	Source of polymerase	Template added	Activity
			pmoles/30 min.
I.	RLV (0.13 unit)	poly(A)·poly(dT)	129
	AMV (0.12 unit)	poly(A)·poly(dT)	122
	AMV + RLV	poly(A)·poly(dT)	252
II.	RLV (0.13 unit)	AMV RNA	0.02
	AMV (0.26 unit)	AMV RNA	1.0
	AMV + RLV	AMV RNA	0.96
III.	RLV (0.2 unit)	[³H]poly(A)·poly(dT)	4
	AMV (0.52 unit)	[³H]poly(A)·poly(dT)	242
	AMV + RLV	[³H]poly(A)·poly(dT)	294

[1] All assays were carried out as described in Methods.

Expt. I.   3.33 nmoles of poly(A), 0.5 nmole of poly(dT), and 1 nmole of [³H]dTTP (794 cpm/pmole) were added to each reaction.

Expt. II.   970 pmoles AMV RNA and 0.8 nmole of α [³²P]dTTP were added to each reaction mixture.

Expt. III.   RNase H activity; 0.87 nmole [³H]poly(A), 30 cpm/pmole and 1 nmole poly(dT) were added to each reaction mixture.

which catalyze adequate RNA-dependent dNMP incorporation (Table 2). In contrast, RNA-directed activity is obtained readily from AMV; mixing of the two purified enzymes resulted in the detection of RNA-dependent dNMP incorporation observed with AMV polymerase alone.

Such preparations of RLV DNA polymerase are also devoid of RNase H activity (Table 2). At present the reason for the discrepancy in the two preparations of polymerase is unclear. We already have noted that there is a molecular weight discrepancy between Rauscher and AMV polymerases as measured by glycerol gradient centrifugation. The former activity is smaller (90,000 vs. 160,000 molecular weight) and may be deficient in a subunit present in the AMV system.

Specificity of action of AMV RNase H

Various homoribopolymers are degraded in the presence of the corresponding complementary homodeoxyribopolymer. These include [³H]poly(A)·poly(dT), [³H]poly(I)·poly(dC), and [³H]poly(C)·poly(dG). In the absence of complementary DNA strands or in the presence of the complementary RNA strands there is virtually no hydrolosis of ribypolymers. An exception to the above is that AMV RNase does not cleave [³H]poly(U)·poly(dA) although this synthetic homopolymer pair is a substrate for *E. coli* RNase (Leis et al., 1973). This specificity of the AMV enzyme is not understood, but it may have important consequences when the enzyme reaches regions rich in uridine. In addition to the synthetic homopolymers listed above, RNA-polymerase products formed with single-stranded circular fd DNA are attacked. The RNA in such hybrid structures was susceptible to digestion (90-95%). The RNase H-resistant RNA was susceptible to digestion by pancreatic RNase in the presence of 0.24 M NaCl.

Products of the reaction

The acid-soluble products released by exhaustive digestion of poly(A)·poly(dT) (95 percent of poly(A) rendered acid-soluble) in the presence of excess AMV RNase H were identified as oligonucleotides (2-8 nucleotides in length) by chromatography of DEAE-cellulose in the presence of urea (Fig. 4). AMP was not detected among the reaction products. The oligoadenylates eluted from the column in the following proportions: di, 22 percent; tri, 8.5 percent; tetra, 12 percent; penta, 15 percent; hexa, 16 percent; hepta, 17 percent; and octa, 9 percent. A similar analysis of digestion products in which 10 percent or 95 percent of the poly(A) rendered acid-

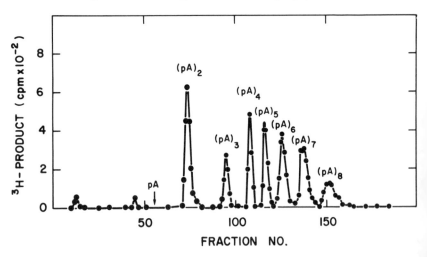

Figure 4.   Separation of acid-soluble degradation products of [³H]poly(A) on DEAE-cellulose in the presence of urea. Procedures for sample preparation are given in Methods.

soluble was made by paper electrophoresis in 0.05 M sodium citrate buffer, pH 3.7. Irrespective of the method of analysis or extent of degradation, all acid-soluble radioactivity generated by RNase H action migrated ahead of [^{14}C] AMP and behind ADP markers simultaneously run as internal standards. No [^{3}H] label co-migrated with the [^{14}C] AMP marker.

The hepta-adenylate peak, isolated after DEAE-cellulose chromatography and dialyzed overnight in the cold against water, was digested to AMP by snake venom phosphodiesterase at pH 9, indicating the presence of 3′ OH termini. Treatment of the unfractionated oligonucleotides with venom diesterase also yielded AMP as the sole product (Baltimore and Smoler, 1972). Treatment of the dialyzed hexa-adenylate peak with bacterial alkaline phosphatase reduced the negative charge of the oligonucleotide, which was detected by a change in electrophoretic migration at pH 3.5. The treated oligonucleotide co-migrated with unlabeled standard (Ap)$_5$A, suggesting that the initial oligonucleotide contained a phosphomonoester terminus. Since the oligonucleotide contains 3′ OH ends, phosphate residues must be at 5′ termini.

Mechanism of action of AMV RNase H

Baltimore and Smoler (1972) recently presented data that AMV RNase H was an endonuclease. This conclusion was based on the observation that [^{32}P] and [^{3}H] from [5′-^{32}P], [3′-^{3}H] doubly labeled poly(A) was rendered acid-soluble almost simultaneously by RNase H action in the presence of poly(dT). We have confirmed these observations, but have demonstrated as previously indicated that RNase H of AMV is in fact a processive exonuclease which acts exonucleolytically in 5′ to 3′ as well as 3′ to 5′ directions (Leis et al, 1973). It is possible to distinguish between these two mechanisms by use of RNA chains without ends. [5′-^{32}P]poly(A) (40 nucleotides long) was treated with T4 RNA ligase, an enzyme that generates circular poly(A) products in which the [^{32}P] is not susceptible to attack by alkaline phosphatase or RNase II. *E. coli* RNase H degrades circular poly(A) to an acid-soluble form in the presence of poly(dT) while AMV RNase H does not (Table 3). Since circular poly(A) has no available ends, we conclude that *E. coli* RNase H is an endonuclease and that the AMV enzyme is an exonuclease.

Table 3.   Influence of substitutions at ends of poly(A) on
the action of RNase H[1]

| Polymer added | Activity (% degradation) by RNase H of | | | |
| | AMV | | E. coli | |
	+Poly(dT)	−Poly(dT)	+Poly(dT)	−Poly(dT)
Circular [^{32}P]poly(A)	<1	<1	81	5
[^{3}H]poly(A)-(dAMP)$_n$	89	0	84	0
[^{3}H]poly(A)-poly(C)·poly(G)	85	0	96	10
Poly(C)-[^{3}H]poly(A)	88	6	95	4
Cellulose-[5′-^{32}P], [^{3}H]poly(A)	75	0	100	0
Cellulose-[5′-^{32}P], [^{3}H]poly(A)-poly(C)·poly(G)	4.6	0	100	4.6

[1] Conditions for RNase H assay given in Methods.

AMV RNase H is a processive exonuclease

A processive nuclease, once bound to a polynucleotide chain, completely degrades the chain before it is released. Thus, if excess [^{3}H]poly(A)·poly(dT) is incubated with a limiting amount of RNase H so that all of the enzyme is bound, the addition of un-labeled poly(A)·poly(dT) to the incubation mixture should have no effect on the acid-solubilization of the labeled poly(A). As shown in Figure 5, the addition of a 16-fold excess of unlabeled poly(A)· poly(dT), 1 minute after the start of the reaction, had no effect on the rate of degradation of [^{3}H]poly(A)·poly(dT) by AMV RNase H. On the other hand, when unlabeled poly(A)·poly(dT) was added to the incubation before RNase H, the rate of [^{3}H]poly(A) degrada-tion was markedly reduced (Fig. 5). This experiment demonstrates that RNase H associated with the AMV RNA-dependent DNA poly-merase acts as a processive exonuclease. In another experiment [^{3}H]poly(A)·poly(dT) was treated with AMV RNase H until 0, 15, and 60 percent of the poly(A) was rendered acid-soluble, then treated with 10 percent formaldehyde (HCHO). Analysis on HCHO-sucrose gradient revealed no large oligonucleotide intermediates. These results also indicate a processive exonuclease activity.

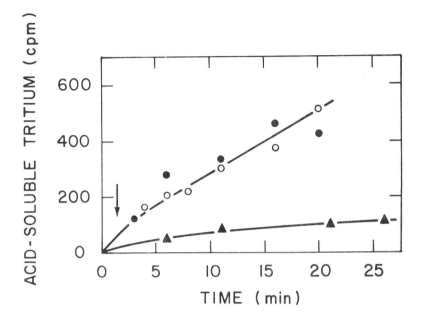

Figure 5.   Effect of adding excess of poly(A)·poly(dT) on the rate of degradation of [³H]poly(A)·poly(dT) by AMV RNase H. Purified AMV RNase H (0.07 unit polymerase, 0.015 unit RNase H) was incubated with [³H]poly(A) (16.9 pmoles, 475 cpm/pmole, prepared with *E. coli* RNA polymerase) and poly(dT) (18.8 pmoles) for various lengths of time. Unlabeled poly(A) (276 pmoles) and poly(dT) (376 pmoles) were added where indicated. AMV RNase H, O——————O; unlabeled poly(A)·poly(dT) added 1 minute after start of incubation (indicated by arrow), ●——————●; unlabeled poly(A)·poly(dT) added before enzyme, △——————△.

Direction of exonucleolytic attack by AMV RNase H

Since AMV RNase H requires ends of RNA chains for activity, we investigated the direction of attack by modifying each end of poly(A) and determining the effect of such modifications on poly(A) degradation. The 3′-hydroxyl end of [³H]poly(A) was blocked by addition of dAMP residues, or by extension of the poly(A) chain with poly(C). In both cases, poly(A) chains that were not extended were removed by digestion with RNase II. Both templates were rendered acid-soluble in the presence of poly(dT) and AMV RNase H (Table 3). The 5′ end of poly(A) was blocked by covalently linking it to cellulose (Leis et al., 1973). Forty-five percent of the covalently linked poly(A) (relative to the amount released by RNase

II) was released by AMV RNase H (Table 3). The 5′ end of poly(A) was also blocked by synthesis of poly(C)-[³H]poly(A) with polynucleotide phosphorylase. The [³H]poly(A) in this polymer was rendered acid-soluble by AMV RNase H. These results indicate that AMV RNase H preparations act in both 5′ to 3′ and 3′ to 5′ directions. Consistent with the above conclusion is the observation that the [³²P] and [³H] from [5′-³²P], [3′-³H]poly(A) were released at the same rate, even when a large molar excess of AMV RNase H to ends of poly(A) was present. The experiment with the circular poly(A) indicated that free ends were required for the reaction. The observation that linkage of the 3′ OH end of cellulose-[5′-³²P]poly(A) to poly(C) prevented degradation of the poly(A) by AMV RNase H in the presence of poly(dT) (Table 3) confirmed the above conclusion. *E. coli* RNase H, an endonuclease, degraded all poly(A) derivatives tested in the presence of poly(dT) (Table 3).

Requirement for duplex hybrid structure for RNase H activity

Mölling and co-workers (1971) reported that the degradation of RNA in RNA-DNA hybrids formed with [³²P] 60S AMV RNA, [³H] deoxynucleotides, and reverse transcriptase exceeded the amount of DNA synthesized during the reaction. This observation suggested that hybrid structures may be required only to initiate degradation but may not be required for continual RNase H activity. We investigated this problem by studying the degradation of [³H]poly(A), after removal of poly(dT) from the incubation mixture, by action of pancreatic DNase. The addition of DNase at any time resulted in an immediate cessation of [³H]poly(A) degradation (Fig. 6). These results indicate that hybrid structures are essential for continued RNase H activity. We also have examined the effect of AMV RNase H on [³²P] Rous sarcoma virus (RSV) RNA during transcription by reverse transcriptase virus (Table 4). The labeled RSV RNA used for these experiments was isolated from virus harvested every 2 hours. With this RNA as primer, deoxynucleotide incorporation represented only 2 percent of the amount of RNA added. Under these conditions there was no extensive deoxynucleotide-dependent acid-solubilization of [³²P] RSV RNA after 50 minutes (approximately 2 pmoles), and this was less than the amount of DNA synthesis that occurred. The precise quantity of DNA was too small to be measured accurately.

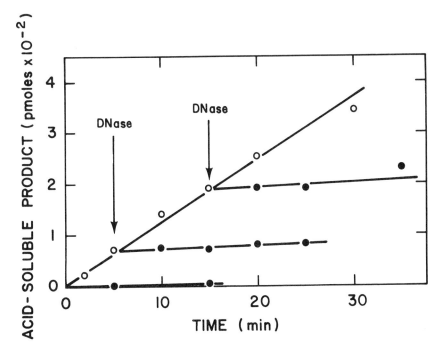

Figure 6.   Effect of addition of pancreatic DNase on RNase H activity. Purified AMV polymerase (0.19 unit) was incubated with [³H]poly(A) (9 cpm/pmole, 1 nmole) and poly(dT) (0.57 nmole) as described in Methods. Pancreatic DNase (5 μg) was added to the incubation mixture at times 0, 5, or 10 minutes after addition of the AMV polymerase as indicated by the arrows. RNase H, O———O; RNase H activity after addition of DNase, ●———●.

Model for tumor virus RNA replication

The extent of RSV RNA-dependent DNA synthesis is limited (Table 4). This observation is also true when 60S AMV RNA is used as primer-template. The limited extent of DNA synthesis might be related to the fact that the polymerase cannot transcribe through extended single-stranded regions of a template and that the 60S RNA is a complex composed of 35S RNA and smaller segments hydrogen-bonded in a partly duplex structure (Bader and Steck, 1969; Cheung et al., 1972; Canaani et al., 1973). The size of the DNA products synthesized is small, as indicated by alkaline sucrose gradient analysis (Fig. 3) and by label transfer experiments (Leis and Hurwitz, 1972b). Furthermore, isopycnic banding in Cs₂SO₄

Table 4.   Simultaneous examination of DNA synthesis
and RNA degradation with AMV polymerase[1]

Time	[32P] RSV RNA remaining			Incorporation of deoxynucleotides
	Omit dNTP	With dNTP	Omit enzyme	
min		*pmoles*		*pmoles*
5	153	155	------	0.96
10	156	156	161	1.04
15	154	152	------	------
20	153	154	154	1.32
30	144	143	151	2.04
40	141	139	148	2.16
50	145	143	147	2.88

[1] Purified AMV polymerase (0.57 unit polymerase, 0.21 unit RNase H) and stimulatory protein (22 ng) were incubated with 157 pmo'es [32P] RSV RNA (32 cpm/pmole) in the presence or absence of deoxynucleotides (label in [3H]dCTP, 100 cpm/pmole) as described in Methods for various lengths of time and acid-insoluble radioactivity measured. Acid-soluble [32P] could not be measured due to the presence of [3H]dCTP.

after formaldehyde denaturation shows covalent attachment of the newly synthesized DNA to RNA primer 3′ OH ends. Since RNA segmented 60 to 70S has a number of such 3′ OH ends, the action of RNA-dependent DNA polymerase on this RNA would generate short covalently linked DNA segments as RNA-DNA hybrids throughout the RNA (Fig. 7) instead of the viral length DNA expected for replication.

The following model for tumor virus replication takes into account all of the known biochemical properties of reverse transcriptase. DNA synthesis could occur with the virus RNA from available 3′ OH ends as shown in Figure 7. The resultant hybrid structure would be susceptible to RNase H cleavage only at each 5′ RNA end and the product of such cleavage would be a RNA-DNA hybrid structure containing single-stranded DNA ends. Such structures, containing single-stranded DNA ends, could possibly be integrated into the host chromosomes and eventually covalently linked through action of DNA ligase. Once integrated, the remaining RNA sequences could be converted into DNA by action of the cellular RNase H (an endonuclease) (Keller and Crouch, 1972) as well as by the nuclear DNA repair machinery. This model predicts that re-

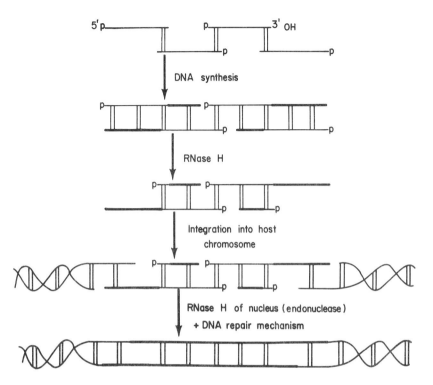

Figure 7.   Postulated role of RNA-dependent DNA polymerase and RNase H in virus replication. Thin lines represent viral RNA, thick lines represent newly synthesized DNA, and the helical structure represents the host chromosome.

verse transcriptase does not completely transcribe viral RNA into DNA as an obligatory step before integration and it predicts that viral RNA sequences can be found in nuclei of infected cells covalently linked to cellular DNA. This model also obviates the necessity to integrate multiple small pieces of viral DNA into the host chromosome.

Distribution of [³H]-UMP RSV RNA in infected cells

To test this model, chick embryo fibroblast (CEF) cells (C/O) were infected with [³H] uridine-labeled RSV (Prague strain, subgroup C, grown on C/O cells and harvested every two hours), and at various times after virus infection cell nuclei and cytoplasmic fractions were prepared. The nucleic acid in each fraction was isolated by a modification of the Penman phenol-SDS method (1966) and analyzed by isopycnic banding in Cs_2SO_4. Averaging the results of two experiments where cell fractions were prepared from 2 to 2.6×10^8 cells 6 hours after infection with [³H] RSV, 89 percent of the radioactivity (4.7×10^6 cpm) was recovered in the cytoplasmic fraction while 11 percent of the label (5.2×10^5 cpm) was recovered in the nuclear fraction. Of the label recovered in the cytoplasmic fraction, 90 percent banded at the density of free RNA in Cs_2SO_4 after heat treatment at 100 C for 3 minutes. The remaining radioactivity was distributed throughout the hybrid and DNA density regions without forming a distinct peak. When the latter material was isolated, dialyzed, heated at 100 C for 2 minutes or 65 C for 15 minutes in the presence of 3 percent HCHO, and then rebanded in Cs_2SO_4, the label now banded as free RNA. These results indicate that the label isolated from the cytoplasmic fraction does not contain stable covalent RNA-DNA structures.

A different distribution of radioactivity was observed from material isolated from nuclei. In experiments with 2×10^7 cells, a kinetic analysis of the [³H] RSV RNA associated with the nuclear fraction was made; [³H] recovered increased with time; for example, radioactivity recovered from nuclei 2, 4, 8, and 10 hours after infection was 6,160, 15,240, 21,400, and 35,900 cpm, respectively. The label at 2 and 4 hours was 87 percent sensitive to alkali treatment (1 M KOH, 7 min. at 100 C), at 8 hours 82 percent was sensitive to alkali, and at 10 hours 67 percent was sensitive to alkaline hydrolysis, suggesting that some RNA label was metabolized to DNA. The radioactivity isolated from nuclei of cells infected for 2 and 4 hours was combined; this material was subjected to isopycnic banding in Cs_2CO_4 before denaturation. The distribution of radioactivity in the gradient was as follows: RNA region, 56 percent; hybrid region (density 1.6-1.5), 9 percent; DNA region, 34 percent. If this material were initially treated with 3 percent HCHO at 65 C for 15 minutes to disrupt hydrogen-bonded secondary structure, the distribution of radioactivity was: RNA region, 50 percent; hybrid region, 32 percent; DNA region, 18 percent. The labeled RNA banding in the hybrid region after denaturation represents RNA covalently linked to unlabeled DNA, and the increase in radioactivity with the concomitant decrease of label in the DNA region indicates that the RNA-DNA hybrid was associated with large amounts of DNA before denaturation. The [³H] recovered in the DNA region after denaturation is contained in RNA.[1] Similar results were obtained with the radioactivity isolated from nuclei 6 to 8 hours and 10 hours after infection.

As the length of time after infection increased, the amount of radioactivity recovered (after denaturation) as hybrid decreased, while the [3H] recovered as DNA increased. The label in the hybrid region at 2 to 4 hours, 6 to 8 hours, and 10 hours was 31, 28, and 18 percent, respectively; the radioactivity recovered in the DNA region after the same time intervals was 18, 25, and 38 percent, respectively.

Properties of isolated RNA-DNA hybrid

The nuclear RNA-DNA covalent hybrid can be isolated without HCHO treatment by sequential heat denaturation and repetitive Cs_2SO_4 banding (at least 2 times) (Fig. 8). The label isolated in the hybrid region (density 1.57) was still in RNA, since it was completely sensitive to RNase digestion and insensitive to DNase (7%). If the RNA-DNA covalent hybrid was heated at 100 C for 2 minutes and then banded for the third time, it still banded at a density of 1.57. Treatment of the hybrid with DNase resulted in a shift of its banding density to 1.61. The labeled RNA recovered from the Cs_2SO_4 gradient banding at 1.61 was hybridized to an excess [32P] dTMP-labeled DNA prepared from RVS by reverse transcriptase. Of the labeled RNA, 55 percent was hybridized to the transcript DNA as measured by its resistance to nuclease S_1, an enzyme specific for single-stranded structures. Furthermore, when analyzed by banding in assay in Cs_2CO_4, the nuclease material resistant to S_1 banded in the hybrid region, which suggests that a substantial portion of the RNA in the RNA-DNA covalent hybrid represents viral RNA sequences.

The RNA of the isolated nuclear RNA-DNA covalent hybrids possessed single-stranded structure since it was completely susceptible to attack by nuclease S_1. The RNA in two different preparations of RNA-DNA covalent hybrids was attacked by RNase II to an ex-

---

[1] The radioactivity recovered in the DNA region by this procedure represents labeled DNA since it bands at a density of 1.46, is 91 percent sensitive to DNase digestion, and 89 percent resistant to RNase. Exhaustive digestion of this material with snake venom diesterase and pancreatic DNase liberated [3H] dCMP as analyzed by paper chromatography in (NH_4OH:isopropanol:borate) and paper electrophoresis at pH 3.5. Thus it appears that some of the labeled viral RNA was degraded to ribomononucleotides, reduced to deoxynucleotides, and utilized for DNA synthesis.

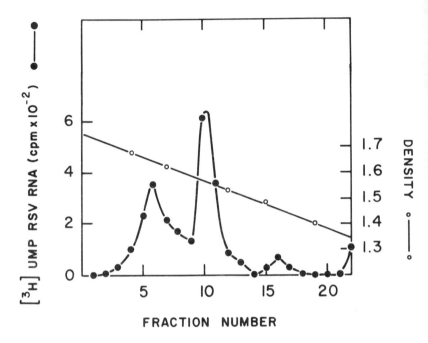

Figure 8.   Isolation of nuclear RNA-DNA covalent hybrids from [³H]uridine-labeled RSV infected cells. Details of the isolation procedure given in Methods.

tent of 23 and 40 percent. RNase II is an exonuclease which attacks RNA from the 3′ end, and it will not attack RNA structures with deoxynucleotides linked at this end. This observation suggests that the formation of RNA-DNA covalent hybrid was not solely due to reverse transcriptase action since the latter system will covalently link DNA only to the 3′ OH end of RNA primers. However, at present, we do not know the source of the DNA present in the RNA-DNA covalent hybrid isolated from nuclei. Experiments are now in progress to isolate DNA covalently linked to viral RNA in order to determine if its origin is cellular, viral, or both.

METHODS

Measurement of RNase H activity

    Reaction mixtures (0.05 ml) containing 1 μmole Tris·HCl, pH 8.0, 0.5 μmole MgCl₂, 0.3 μmole dithioerythritol, 2μg bovine serum albumin, 0.52 nmole poly(dT), 0.56 nmole [³H]poly(A), and AMV polymerase or *E. coli* RNase H were incubated for 30 minutes at 38 C. Reactions were stopped by addition of 0.1 ml of a solution containing sodium pyrophosphate, 0.4 mg albumin, 52 nmoles denatured salmon sperm DNA, and 0.5 ml 5 percent trichloroacetic acid. The reaction mixtures were centrifuged at 2,000 rpm in an International centrifuge and the supernatant collected and counted in 10 ml of Bray's scintillation fluid.

Measurement of viral polymerase activity

Unless otherwise indicated, the reaction mixtures for AMV RNA-directed DNA synthesis (0.05 ml) contained 1 μmole of Tris·HCl, pH 8.0, 0.5 μmole of $MgCl_2$, 0.25 μmole of KCl, 0.3 μmole of dithioerythritol, 5 nmoles each of dATP, dGTP, dCTP, labeled dTTP, AMV, RNA, purified RLV polymerase or purified AMV polymerase. Poly(A)·poly(dT)-directed DNA synthesis was measured in an identical manner except that virus RNA, dATP, dGTP, and dCTP were omitted. The amounts of enzyme and labeled deoxyribonucleoside triphosphate are given in the tables.

Reactions were stopped after 30 minutes incubation at 38 C by the addition of 0.1 ml of 0.1 M sodium pyrophosphate, 0.02 ml of denatured salmon sperm DNA (2.6 μmoles/ml), and 5 percent trichloroacetic acid. After 5 minutes at 4 C, acid-insoluble material was collected on Gelman type E glass fiber filters, dried, and counted in 10 ml of toluene scintillation fluid in a scintillation spectrometer.

RNase H assay of modified poly(A)

Poly(A), modified as described (Leis et al., 1973), was treated as follows:

1. Circular [³²P]poly(A) (2,000 cpm, 0.35 nmole)·poly(dT) (1 nmole) was incubated with purified AMV polymerase (0.4 unit polymerase, 0.1 unit RNase H) and stimulatory protein (22.8 ng) or *E. coli*. RNase H (0.66 unit) for 30 minutes at 38 C; acid-insoluble radioactivity was determined as described (Leis and Hurwitz, 1972b).

2. [³H]poly(A)-(dAMP)ₙ (14.1 pmole, 32 cpm/pmole) was incubated with or without poly(dT) (0.25 nmole) with either AMV RNase H (0.38 unit polymerase, 0.084 unit RNase H) or *E. coli* RNase H (0.44 unit) for 30 minutes at 38 C, as described in step 1.

3. [³H]poly(A)-poly(C)·poly(G) (129 pmole, 9 cpm/pmole) was incubated with or without poly(dT) (1 nmole) with either AMV RNase H (0.38 unit polymerase, 0.084 unit RNase H) and

stimulatory protein (17 ng) or *E. coli* RNase H (0.44 unit) for 30 minutes at 38 C.

4. Poly(C)-[^{3}H]poly(A) (141 pmole, 9 cpm/pmole) was incubated with or without poly(dT) (0.2 nmole) with either AMV RNase H (0.38 unit polymerase, 0.084 unit RNase H) and stimulatory protein (17 ng) or *E. coli* RNase H (0.44 unit) for 30 minutes at 38 C.

5. A suspension (0.1 ml) of cellulose-[5′-^{32}P], [^{3}H]poly(A) (1,800 cpm [^{3}H], 9 cpm/pmole) was centrifuged at 3,000 rpm for 2 minutes in an International centrifuge, and the supernatant was discarded. The cellulose was suspended in a reaction mixture (0.05 ml) containing AMV RNase H (1.9 units polymerase, 0.42 unit RNase H) and stimulatory protein (17 ng) or *E. coli* RNase H (3.3 units) with or without poly(dT) (2 nmole); tubes were mixed every 5 minutes during the incubation. After 60 minutes at 38 C, the reaction was stopped by the addition of 0.2 ml of cold water and centrifuged in an International centrifuge for 2 minutes at 3,000 rpm. The supernatant was counted in 10 ml of Bray's scintillation fluid. The cellulose was suspended in 0.2 ml of water and also counted in 10 ml of Bray's scintillation fluid. The amount of poly(A) released from the cellulose by RNase II was assumed to be all of the poly(A) accessible to attack by a processive nuclease.

6. Cellulose-[5′^{32}P], [^{3}H]poly(A)-poly(C)·poly(G) (1,320 cpm [^{3}H], 9 cpm/pmole) was treated as described in step 5.

Isolation of DNA product and centrifugation in sucrose gradient

Protein was extracted from each reaction mixture containing DNA products with 0.5 ml phenol (neutralized and saturated with water) and the deproteinized mixtures were dialyzed for 2 hours at 4 C against 500 ml of a solution containing 0.3 M NaCl and 0.03 M sodium citrate. Twenty μmoles EDTA was added to each dialyzed fraction and RNA was hydrolyzed with 0.7 N NaOH overnight at 38 C. The recovery of acid-insoluble radioactivity was 9,540 cpm (in 0.6 ml) and 46,800 cpm (in 0.7 ml) for the mixtures lacking and containing stimulatory protein, respectively. Aliquots of these mixtures containing 4,760 and 11,300 cpm were layered over a 5 ml 5 to 20 percent sucrose gradient in 0.7 M NaCl, 0.3 N NaOH, and 5 mM EDTA and centrifuged at 50,000 rpm at 20 C for 140 minutes in a Spinco SW 50.1 rotor. *E. coli* virus [^{14}C] fd DNA was included in the gradient as a marker. Thirty fractions were collected, precipitated with trichloroacetic acid, collected on glass fiber filters, dried, and counted in toluene scintillation fluid in a scintillation counter under double-label counting conditions. The spill of [^{32}P] into [^{14}C] channel was 4 percent; [^{14}C] into [^{32}P] was 0.5 percent and counting efficiency of [^{32}P] was 69 percent of normal counting efficiency. Recovery of [^{32}P] label from the sucrose gradients was 80 to 90 percent.

Analysis of degradation products of [^{3}H]poly(A) by RNase H

Reaction mixtures (0.3 ml) containing purified AMV polymerase (0.88 unit), stimulatory protein (19 ng), [^{3}H]poly(A) (32 cpm/pmole, 4.33 nmoles), and poly(dT) (6.5 nmoles) were incubated under conditions described in Table 1. After 60 minutes at 38 C, 95 percent of the poly(A) was rendered acid-soluble; the reaction was stopped by the addition of 2 μmoles of EDTA, 0.8 mg of albumin, 0.1 μmole of denatured salmon sperm DNA, and 0.5 ml of 5 percent trichloracetic acid. An identical second incubation with unlabeled poly(A) (32 nmoles) was treated in a similar fashion and added to the first as carrier. After centrifugation for 5 minutes at 3,000 rpm in an International centrifuge, the supernatant containing 1.01 x 10^5 cpm was extracted four times with three volumes of ether and dried *in vacuo*. The residue was dissolved in 4 ml of a solution containing 0.02 M Tris·HCl, pH 7.5, and 7 M urea (buffer A) and applied to a 0.5 x 110 cm DEAE-cellulose column equilibrated with buffer A at room temperature. The column was developed with a 600 ml linear sodium chloride gradient (0-0.6 M in buffer A) at a flow rate of 16 ml/hr. Two ml fractions were collected and aliquots (0.5 ml) were counted in 10 ml of Bray's scintillation fluid. The recovery of [^{3}H] was quantitative. (The radioactivities plotted in Fig. 4 are the actual counts of aliquots, uncorrected for quenching. To obtain total cpm/sample, corrected for quenching, each sample should be multiplied by 8.84.)

Procedure for isolating RNA-DNA covalent hybrids from cells infected with [^{3}H] uridine-labeled Rous sarcoma virus

Rous sarcoma virus (Prague, subgroup C) was grown on chick embryo fibroblast monolayers (C/O cells). Virus was labeled by incubating infected cells 12 to 15 hours with 10 mCi of [^{3}H] uridine (2 x 10^4 cpm/pmole)/60 ml growth medium (Cheung et al., 1972). After this period, the growth medium was removed and the cells washed twice with unlabeled growth medium; washed cells were

COLORADO COLLEGE LIBRARY
COLORADO SPRINGS,
COLORADO

then incubated with 50 ml of growth medium and virus harvested at 2 to 3 hour intervals. Cells were removed by centrifugation at 800 xg for 10 minutes and the supernatant, containing virus (5 x 10⁶ FFU/ ml), was used to infect cells. Chick embryo fibroblasts (CEF), primary cultures (C/O) grown to confluency (4 days past seeding), were trypsinized and seeded at 20 x 10⁶ cells/25 ml into 150 x 25 mm petri dishes. After 3 hours incubation at 37 C in a 5 percent CO_2 humidified atmosphere, each plate was treated with 5 ml of labeled virus suspension containing unlabeled uridine (2 x 10⁻⁶ M). After 30 minutes, fresh growth medium was added and cells were incubated for 6 hours. Monolayers were washed and trypsinized (0.25% trypsin for 1 min.), and cells were suspended in growth medium and pelleted at 400 xg for 5 minutes. Cells were washed twice and then resuspended in a solution containing 0.01 M Tris·HCl, pH 7.4, 0.01 M NaCl, and 1.5 mM $MgCl_2$ (RSB) at a concentration of 2 to 4 x 10⁷ cells/ml. After 15 minutes on ice, cells were gently homogenized 5 to 10 times in a tight-fitting homogenizer in 1 percent Tween 40 and 0.5 percent DOC. Nuclei were pelleted at 800 xg for 2.5 minutes, suspended in 2 ml of RSB containing the detergent, pelleted, and frozen at –20 C. The supernatant obtained after pelleting of nuclei was used to isolate cytoplasmic nuclei acid fractions. Such supernatants were adjusted to 0.01 M EDTA and 1 percent SDS and treated with 2 volumes of 95 percent ethanol. After centrifugation, pellets were dissolved in a solution containing 0.5 percent SDS, 0.01 M Tris·HCl, pH 7.4, 0.01 M NaCl, and 1 mM EDTA and frozen. Nuclear fractions contained 1.65 x 10⁵ acid-insoluble cpm, while cytoplasmic fractions contained 3.71 x 10⁶ acid-insoluble cpm.

Nucleic acid was extracted from nuclei and cytoplasmic fractions by a modification of the Penman procedure (1966). Nuclear fractions were suspended in 0.8 ml of a solution containing 0.5 percent SDS, 50 mM EDTA and treated with 1 volume of phenol (neutralized and saturated with water) at 60 C for 2 minutes. Phases were mixed with a Vortex mixer for 20 seconds. One volume of 1 percent isoamyl alcohol in chloroform was added and the mixture was incubated at 60 C for 2 minutes. After centrifugation, the phenol-chloroform phase was removed and the aqueous phase was extracted three times, each with an equal volume of 1 percent isoamyl alcohol in chloroform at 25 C. The aqueous phase (1.3 ml) containing 1.59 x 10⁵ cpm was collected and adjusted to 10 mM EDTA, 25 mM sodium phosphate pH 7 and heated at 100 C for 3 minutes and then placed in ice. The cooled solution was treated with 0.4 ml of 10 x SSC and 0.01 ml of 10 percent sarkosyl and the mixture diluted to 4 ml. Solid Cs_2SO_4 (2.8 g) was added, yielding a refractive index of 1.3780, and the mixture was centrifuged for 67 hours at 32,000 rpm in a Spinco SW65 rotor at 22 C. Eighteen drop fractions were collected from a hole pierced in the bottom of the tube and refractive indices were determined. Tritium label was distributed as follows: RNA region (density 1.69-1.63), 39,550 cpm; hybrid region (density 1.63-1.49), 66,300 cpm; DNA region (density 1.49-1.43), 28,575 cpm. The material banding between the density of 1.63 and 1.49 was pooled and dialyzed overnight at 4 C against 1 l of 10 mM sodium phosphate pH 7 and 1 mM EDTA, brought to a final volume of 4 ml containing 35 mM sodium phosphate pH 7, 11 mM EDTA, 0.025 percent sarkosyl, heated to 100 C for 3 minutes and cooled in ice. Cs_2SO_4 was added as above and the mixture was centrifuged at 30,000 rpm in a Spinco SW 50.1 rotor at 20 C for 64 hours. Fractions were collected as above, refractive indices measured, and 0.01 ml aliquots precipitated with TCA and counted. Recovery of label from the Cs_2SO_4 gradient was >85 percent.

Tritium-labeled RSV RNA, ●————●; density, ○————○.

DISCUSSION

The presence of RNase H activity associated with purified AMV reverse transcriptase has been reported by several laboratories Mölling et al., 1971; Baltimore and Smoler, 1972; Grandgenett et al., 1972; Keller and Crouch, 1973; Leis et al., 1973; Watson et al., 1973). This nuclease activity degrades a variety of ribhomopolymers, with the exception of poly(U), in the presence of their complementary deoxyribohomopolymers including natural RNA in fd DNA-RNA hybrid structures. The products of degradation of poly(A)·poly(dT) are oligonucleotides 2 to 8 adenylate residues in length containing 5′ phosphate and 3′ OH termini. Similar observations have been reported by Baltimore and Smoler (1972) and Keller and Crouch 1972).

RNase H activity has been reported to co-chromatograph with reverse transcriptase during purification (Mölling et al., 1971; Baltimore and Smoler, 1972; Keller and Crouch, 1972; Watson et al., 1973; Grandgenett et al., 1972). However, when AMV reverse transcriptase is purified in our laboratory by phosphocellulose chromatography, small and occasionally variable chromatographic differences are observed between DNA polymerase and RNase H activities. The active catalytic sites for polymerase and nuclease activities may be different since they possess different sensitivities to heat or NEM. At present, however, we have been unsuccessful in separating polymerase free of RNase H and therefore cannot distinguish whether the two activities are part of a single enzyme molecule composed of different subunits or different enzyme molecules that co-chromatograph during purification. Our data do not fit completely with the observations reported by Grandgenett and co-workers (1972) that AMV reverse transcriptase is composed of a single polypeptide chain of 70,000 molecular weight containing RNase H and DNA polymerase activities. Of the other purified reverse transcriptases examined, only RSV polymerase has RNase H activity. Rauscher leukemia virus DNA polymerase, which catalyzes both d(AT) copolymer and poly(A)·poly(dT)-directed incorporation lacks RNase H activity. This lack of detectable activity is not due to an inhibitor or a contaminating nucleolytic activity since mixing RLV and AMV polymerase preparations does not inhibit AMV RNase H activity. The RLV polymerase also lacks detectable 60S viral (AMV, RLV, RSV) RNA-dependent DNA polymerase activity. Similar observations have been made by Gallo and co-workers (pers. comm.), Scolnick and co-workers (pers. comm.), and Duesberg and co-workers (pers. comm.). The molecular weight of this polymerase has been estimated at 90,000 by glycerol gradient centrifugation. Tronick and co-workers (1972) have determined a molecular weight of 70,000 by gel filtration. Since purified AMV polymerase has a molecular weight of 160,000, a subunit of the RLV polymerase responsible for RNA-primed DNA synthesis and perhaps RNase H activity may have been lost during its purification.

The AMV RNase H has been shown to be a processive exonuclease (Leis et al., 1973). The nuclease has an absolute requirement for ends of RNA chains for activity, as shown by its inability to digest circular poly(A) or poly(A) blocked at both 3' and 5' ends. Furthermore, the rate of degradation [^{3}H]poly(A)·poly(dT) is unaffected by the addition of excess unlabeled poly(A)·poly(dT) after start of the reaction. These results can be explained if AMV RNase H acts as a processive exonuclease. The exonucleolytic cleavage can occur in both 5' to 3' and 3' to 5' directions, as shown by the ability of the nuclease preparation to degrade poly(A) blocked either at the

5′ or 3′ ends. Evidence that AMV RNase H is not an endonuclease also was presented by Keller and Crouch (1972), who demonstrated that AMV RNase H did not attack polyribonucleotides of unknown chain length contained in a heterogenous population of colicin E1 circular duplex DNA.

The fact that the AMV RNase H is a processive exonuclease which requires ends of RNA chains for activity suggests it has a limited effect on viral RNA during transcription. There should be no attack of viral RNA until an RNA end in RNA-DNA hybrid structure is generated during transcription. Internal RNA-DNA hybrids should not be susceptible to attack. When [^{32}P] RSV RNA was incubated with purified preparations of AMV reverse transcriptase under conditions in which deoxynucleotide incorporation represents 2 percent of the RNA added, there was little detectable dNTP acid-solubilization of the [^{32}P] label. This observation is in contrast to that reported by Mölling and co-workers (1971), where hydrolysis of AMV RNA greatly exceeded the amount of RNA-DNA hybrid synthesized during the reaction. The requirement for hybrid structure for active RNase H activity is clearly demonstratable with [^{3}H]poly(A)·poly(dT). The removal of poly(dT) at any time during the reaction by DNase digestion halts the degradation of the [^{3}H]poly(A) immediately.

The action of AMV RNase H on RNA-primed DNA transcripts would be to specifically remove RNA from both 5′ phosphate ends generating single-stranded DNA regions. These single-stranded DNA ends could be used by the host cell recombination machinery to incorporate the hybrid structure directly into the host chromosome. In this way, it may not be necessary to transcribe all RNA regions into DNA before integration. Once this structure is integrated, RNase H of the nucleus (an endonuclease, Keller and Crouch, 1972) could remove internally situated RNA hybrid structures and the host DNA-repair machinery could convert these structures into DNA. This mechanism would obviate the necessity to integrate multiple small pieces of DNA into the host chromosome. A diagrammatic summary of the postulated reaction is presented in Figure 7.

The mechanism proposed in Figure 7 predicts that after infection, integration of part of the oncornaviral RNA into the host chromosome will occur. In addition, it suggests that RNA-dependent DNA polymerase may be responsible for converting viral RNA of suitable structure (partly duplex in structure, with a primer-template relationship) into RNA-DNA hybrids, rather than catalyzing the transcription of the entire RNA genome into DNA.

The mechanism of virus RNA replication is unknown. Since the genetic information of the virus proposed above would reside within the host chromosome, a second prediction of this model is that the synthesis of oncornaviral RNA is catalyzed by the DNA-dependent RNA polymerase of the host.

We have begun a search for viral RNA directly integrated into the host chromosome (covalently linked to cellular DNA) as would be predicted if integration occurs before complete transcription to DNA. Experiments in progress have indicated that Prague RSV RNA ([3H]-uridine labeled) can be recovered specifically in the nucleus of infected CEF (C/O) cells covalently linked to DNA. The viral RNA-DNA covalent hybrid is not detected in cytoplasmic cell fractions, suggesting that there is something unique in the tumor RNA replication pathway that requires interaction of the infecting virus and the nucleus of the cell. Whether this interaction is involved in uncoating the virus or providing a necessary factor(s) for transcription is unknown.

The isolation of a viral RNA-DNA covalent hybrid in the nucleus of infected cells does not provide proof that viral RNA sequences have been integrated, since such a hybrid could be generated by reverse transcriptase action. However, the association of the viral RNA-DNA covalent hybrid with large amounts of DNA before denaturation and the observations that RNA in the covalent hybrid is partially sensitive to RNase II suggest the presence of structures in which RNA exists at 3' ends with DNA either internally located or at 5' end (or both). Some of the viral RNA sequences may be covalently linked to cellular DNA as predicted by the model. Experiments are now in progress to label the DNA covalently linked to the viral RNA, isolate it, and identify its origin by direct hybridization.

Acknowledgments: We thank Robert Santini for excellent technical assistance, J. Beard for generous gifts of AMV, and R. Smith for helpful discussion on growing chick embryo fibroblasts.

This work was supported by grants from the Special Viral Cancer Program of the National Institutes of Health (71-2251); National Institutes of Health (GM-13344), National Institutes of Health (5 SO4 RR 06148), and the American Cancer Society (NP-89-1). J. P. Leis is a fellow of the Damon Runyon Cancer Foundation (DRF-659). A. L. Schincariol is a fellow of the National Cancer Institute of Canada.

Literature Cited

Alberts, B. M. 1967. Fractionation of nucleic acids by dextran-polyethylene glycol two-phase system. In *Methods in Enzymology*, Vol. XII, Part A. L. Grossman and K. Moldave, eds., pp. 556-581. New York: Academic Press.

Bader, J. 1964. The role of deoxyribonucleic acid in the synthesis of Rous sarcoma virus. Virology, *22:* 462-468.

Bader, J. P., and T. L. Steck. 1969. Analysis of the ribonucleic acid of murine leukemia virus. J. Virol, *4:*454-459.

Baltimore, D. 1970. RNA-dependent DNA polymerase in virions of RNA tumor viruses. Nature (London), *226:* 1209-1211.

Baltimore, D., and D. Smoler. 1972. Association of an endonuclease with the avian myeloblastosis virus DNA polymerase. J. Biol. Chem., *247:* 7282-7287.

Canaani, E., K. Helm, and P. Duesberg. 1973. Evidence for 30-40S RNA as precursor of the 60-70S RNA from Rous sarcoma virus. Proc. Nat. Acad. Sci. U.S., *70:* 401-405.

Cheung, K. S., R. E. Smith, M. P. Stone, and K. W. Joklik. 1972. Comparison of immature (rapid harvest) and mature Rous sarcoma virus particles. Virology, *50:* 851-864.

Duesberg, P., K. V. D. Helm, and E. Canaani. 1971. Comparative properties of RNA and DNA templates for the DNA polymerase of Rous sarcoma virus. Proc. Nat. Acad. Sci. U.S., *68:* 2505-2509.

Grandgenett, D. P., G. F. Gerard, and M. Green. 1972. Ribonuclease H: A ubiquitous activity in virions of ribonucleic acid tumor viruses. J. Virol., 1136-1142.

Hurwitz, J., and J. Leis. 1972. RNA-dependent DNA polymerase activity of RNA tumor viruses. I. Directing influence of DNA in the reaction. J. Virol., *9:* 116-129.

Kacian, D., K. Watson, A. Burny, and S. Spiegelman. 1971. Purification of the DNA polymerase of avian myeloblastosis virus. Biochim. Biophys. Acta, *246:* 365-383.

Keller, W., and R. Crouch. 1972. Degradation of DNA-RNA hybrids of ribonuclease H and DNA polymerases of cellular and viral origin. Proc. Nat. Acad. Sci. U.S., *69:* 3360-3364.

Leis, J., I. Berkower, and J. Hurwitz. 1973. Isolation and characterization of an avian myeloblastosis virus stimulatory protein. In *DNA synthesis in vitro*, proceedings of a symposium, Madison, Wisc., July 1972. R. D. Wells and R. B. Inman, eds., pp. 287-308. Baltimore: University Park Press.

Leis, J., I. Berkower, and J. Hurwitz. 1973. Mechanism of action of ribonuclease H isolated from avian myeloblastosis virus, and *Escherichia coli.* Proc. Nat. Acad. Sci. U.S., *70:* 466-470.

Leis, J., and J. Hurwitz. 1972a. RNA-dependent DNA polymerase activity of RNA tumor viruses. II. Directing influence of RNA in the reaction. J. Virol., *9:* 130-142.

Leis, J., and J. Hurwitz. 1972b. Isolation and characterization of a protein that stimulates DNA synthesis from avian myeloblastosis virus. Proc. Nat. Acad. Sci. U.S., 69: 2331-2335.

Mölling, K., D. P. Bolognesi, H. Bauer, W. Büsen, H. W. Plassman, and P. Hausen. 1971. Association of viral reverse transcriptase with an enzyme degrading the RNA moiety of RNA-DNA hybrids. Nature New Biol. 234: 240-243.

Penman, S. 1966. RNA metabolism in the HeLa cell nucleus. J. Mol. Biol. 17: 117-130.

Scolnick, E., E. Rands, S. A. Aaronson, and G. Todaro. 1970. RNA-dependent DNA polymerase activity in five RNA viruses: Divalent cation requirements. Proc. Nat. Acad. Sci. U.S., 67: 1789-1796.

Smoler, D., I. Molineux, and D. Baltimore. 1971. Direction of polymerization by the avian myeloblastosis virus deoxyribonucleic acid polymerase. J. Biol. Chem., 246: 7697-7700.

Spiegelman, S., A. Burny, M. R. Das, J. Keydar, J. Schlom, M. Travnicek, and K. Watson. 1970. Synthetic DNA-RNA hybrids and RNA-DNA duplexes as templates for the polymerase of the oncogenic RNA viruses. Nature (London), 228: 430-432.

Taylor, J. M., A. J. Faras, H. E. Varmus, W. E. Levinson, and J. M. Bishop. 1972. Ribonucleic acid directed deoxyribonucleic acid synthesis by the purified deoxyribonucleic acid polymerase of Rous sarcoma virus. Characterization of the enzymatic product. Biochemistry, 11: 2343-2351.

Temin, H. M. 1964. The participation of DNA in Rous sarcoma virus production. Virology, 23: 486-494.

Temin, H. M., and S. Mizutani. 1970. RNA-dependent DNA polymerase in virions of Rous sarcoma virus. Nature (London), 226: 1211-1213.

Tronick, S. R., E. M. Scolnick, and W. P. Parks. 1972. Reversible inactivation of the deoxyribonucleic acid polymerase of Rauscher leukemia virus. J. Virol. 10: 885-888.

Verma, I. M., N. L. Meuth, E. Bromfield, K. Manly, and D. Baltimore. 1971. A covalently linked RNA-DNA molecule as the initial product of the RNA tumor virus DNA polymerase. Nature New Biol., 233: 131-134.

Vigier, P., and A. Goldé. 1964. Effects of actinomycin D and mitomycin C on the development of Rous sarcoma virus. Virology, 23: 511-519.

Watson, K. F., M. Mölling, and H. Bauer. 1973. Ribonuclease H activity present in purified DNA polymerase from avian myeloblastosis virus. Biochem. Biophys. Res. Commun., 51: 232-240.

The SV40 Genome and Its Transcription

John E. Newbold
*Department of Bacteriology
    and Immunology
School of Medicine
University of North Carolina
Chapel Hill, North Carolina 27514*

Simian virus 40 (SV40) is a small DNA-containing tumor virus whose natural host appears to be monkeys. In the context of viral taxonomy, SV40 and the very similar polyoma virus of mice are among the smallest members of the papovavirus group. Small viruses have traditionally been choice systems for detailed analysis due to their limited complement of genetic information. For the DNA viruses, "small" is used here to denote a genome equivalent to a double-stranded DNA molecule of 2 to 4 x 10^6 daltons. The duplex DNA genomes of SV40 and polyoma viruses are variously estimated to be 3.0 to 3.6 x 10^6 daltons. The other small DNA viruses are the single-stranded DNA phages of *Escherichia coli*, for example ϕx174, S_{13}, fd, and M_{13}, and the parvovirus (or picodnavirus) group, whose genome is likewise single-stranded DNA. The small papovaviruses have become the object of intensive study by molecular biologists in the last decade because they lend themselves conveniently to the study of two important phenomena in the biology of eukaryote cells:

1. Viral transformation. The *in vitro* analog of the initial events in the process of viral tumorigenesis.

2. The metabolism of RNA in eukaryote cells. The transcription of the papovavirus genome in the nucleus of the infected cell, and the subsequent processing of that RNA, seems to mimic the scheme for transcription of the more complex host genome.

At this time a clear understanding of both of the aforementioned phenomena in the papovavirus systems is still not available. Nonetheless, our knowledge of the molecular genetics of the SV40 virus has increased considerably in the past two years, primarily due to the application of site-specific restriction endonucleases. The characterization of the specific-limit fragments of SV40 DNA produced in such digests has generated a physical cleavage map of the viral genome which could serve as a reference for mapping template functions, integration sites, and structural genes of the SV40 chromosome. The studies described in this paper have taken just this approach; namely to dissect the SV40 genome with a site-specific restriction endonuclease, to relate those specific fragments to the physical cleavage map developed for SV40 DNA by Danna, Sack, and Nathans (1973), and to use those specific fragments to probe the composition of the late viral messenger RNA species isolated intact from the cytoplasm of infected cells. These studies are directed at understanding both the general problem of RNA metabolism in eukaryote cells and the mechanism of viral transformation. Transformation may be a consequence of the inability of the infected cell to synthesize the late viral mRNA species and thus to support a productive and cytocidal infection.

Restriction enzymes are DNases which introduce a limited number of cleavages into duplex DNA and at present are isolated only from certain strains of bacteria. The restriction endonucleases can be grouped into two classes, depending upon whether or not the cleavages are specific. In the mapping studies of the SV40 genome, only the site-specific restriction enzymes have been exploited. Table 1 summarizes the sensitivity of SV40 DNA to digestion by several of the site-specific restriction enzymes. An adequate number of specific endonucleases is available to dissect the SV40 genome for a detailed physical analysis. The list given in Table 1 must not be considered complete but can be expected to grow as more bacterial strains are monitored for restriction enzymes. Additionally, the enzymes listed in Table 1 do not all have distinct cleavage specificities. The restriction enzymes *Hinb* and *Hind*III appear to act at identical cleavage sites: the *Hpa* I enzyme has a cleavage specificity that is a subset of the *Hind*II enzyme. The studies described in this paper involve primarily the enzyme *Hae* III from *Hemophilus aegyptius*.

Electrophoresis in cylindrical acrylamide gels of limit digests of SV40 DNA using endonuclease *Hae* III resolves 10 major specific

Table 1.   Sensitivity of SV40 DNA to restriction enzymes

Bacterium	Restriction enzyme[1]	No. of cleavage sites
E. coli RTF RI	*Eco*RI	1
E. coli RTF RII	*Eco*RII	16
H. influenzae, serotype b	*Hin*b	6
H. influenzae, serotype d	*Hin*dII	5
H. influenzae, serotype d	*Hin*dIII	6
H. parainfluenzae	*Hpa* I	3
H. parainfluenzae	*Hpa* II	1
H. aegyptius	*Hae* III	10
Serratia marcescens	*Sma*	0

[1] Using the nomenclature proposed by Smith and Nathans, 1973.

fragments (Huang et al., 1973). As reported previously, differences in the limit fragment pattern can be detected between different independent laboratory strains of SV40 (Huang et al., 1973). Figure 1 shows such data for the Vogt-Dulbecco small plaque strain and the Pagano large plaque strain. The DNA fragments seen in Figure 1 are visualized by fluorescence after staining the extruded gels with the intercalative dye, ethidium bromide. (The Vogt-Dulbecco strain was derived from virus obtained from A.B. Sabin and cloned by M. Vogt. The Pagano strain was obtained from K. Takemoto at N.I.H. and further cloned in J. Pagano's laboratory.) The Vogt-Dulbecco strain shows 10 bands: *Hae* III – A, B, C, D, E, F_1, F_2, X, G, and H; the Pagano strain also shows 10 bands: *Hae* III – A, B, C, D, E_1, E_2, F_1, F_2, G, and H. Limit digests of mixtures of these two virus strains reveal that the *Hae* III-E band of the Vogt-Dulbecco virus shows an electrophoretic mobility identical with the *Hae* III – E_1 band of the Pagano virus. Bands *Hae* III-A, B, C, D, F_1, F_2, G, and H show identical mobilities in the two virus strains. The strain difference is strikingly apparent. The Vogt-Dulbecco virus has a fragment *Hae* III-X with mobility intermediate between *Hae* III-F_2 and *Hae* III-G, which the Pagano virus lacks; the Pagano virus contains the fragment *Hae* III-E_2 which is absent in the Vogt-Dulbecco strain.

Since laboratory strains of SV40 may differ slightly in their limit cleavage patterns and since Danna, Sack, and Nathans (1973) have developed a physical map for SV40 DNA using the *Hind* and *Hpa*

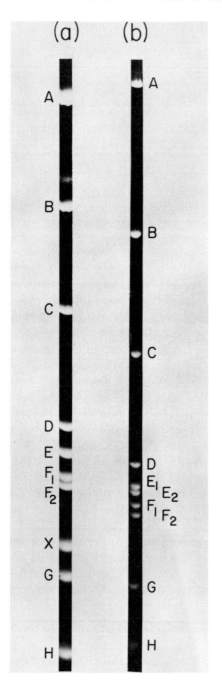

Figure 1. Limit fragment patterns for 10 μg (approx.) SV40 DNA digested by *Hae* III and resolved by electrophoresis on cylindrical polyacrylamide gels: (a) Vogt-Dulbecco virus strain, (b) Pagano strain. DNA fragments are visualized by fluoresence after staining with ethidium bromide. The two photographs are from quite independent analyses and represent gels of different composition, porosity and dimensions. Thus, homologous fragments in the two virus strains show different relative mobilities in this composite photograph. Analysis of DNA fragments derived from a mixture of the two virus strains and fractionated on one gel reveals that bands A, B, C, D, E, F_1, F_2, G and H of gel (a) are homologous with bands, A, B, C, D, E_1, F_1, F_2 G, and H respectively of gel (b). Resolution of band E of the Pagano virus into the components E_1 and E_2 is obtained using very long gels. Gel (a) was 25 cm long, whereas (b) was 60 cm long.

restriction enzymes, it became clear that the Nathans strain of SV40 (small plaque strain 776) would become the standard strain for mapping studies. Limit cleavage of the Nathans virus DNA by *Hae* III enzyme gives a fragment pattern which is distinct from either the Vogt-Dulbecco or Pagano strains. In this digest ten specific fragments are obtained, although only nine bands are resolved . . . one of the bands is represented as a two-molar yield and is considered to be an unresolved doublet. The bands are *Hae* III-A, B, C, D, E, F_1, F_2, G, and H. Band F_1 is the unresolved doublet, denoted as F_{1a} and F_{1b}. As in the Vogt-Dulbecco strain, the *Hae* III-E band of the Nathans virus shows electrophoretic homology with the *Hae* III-E_1 fragment of the Pagano virus.

From this analysis of the three different SV40 strains with the *Hae* III enzyme, it would appear that SV40 DNA is comprised of the nine fragments *Hae* III-A, B, C, D, E_1, F_{1a}, F_2, G, and H. In addition, the viral DNA will contain the fragment E_2 (Pagano strain), F_{1b} (Nathans strain), or X (Vogt-Dulbecco). It is immediately clear that net deletions or insertions of the appropriate size will convert the fragment pattern of one virus strain into either of the other two. At this time it is not known if the DNA fragments *Hae* III-E_2, F_{1b}, and X exhibit any common sequence homology.

If the fragment *Hae* III-X proves to be a specific subfragment of *Hae* III-F_{1b}, which in turn is a specific subfragment of *Hae* III-E_2, then there are interesting consequences regarding the structure and function of the SV40 genome. First, if we can assume that in the *Hae* III cleavage analysis of these three different strains of SV40 that a large number of very small (1-30 base pairs) specific fragments has not been generated, a possibility that has not been carefully monitored in these studies, then we must conclude that the molecular weight of the SV40 DNA varies somewhat from one virus strain to another, being greatest for the Pagano virus and least for the Vogt-Dulbecco strain. Second, and also drawing on the assumption just mentioned, it would appear that the possible variation in size of the SV40 genome is confined predominantly to a single location in the SV40 DNA molecule. The question then immediately arises as to the possibility that this "variable" region of the genome represents informational DNA, i.e., sequences that are transcribed or translated.

The construction of a physical cleavage map for the SV40 genome requires two determinations: the size of each of the limit fragments and the relative order of the different limit fragments. In our previous studies of *Hae* III digestion of SV40 DNA, fragment sizes were measured by coelectrophoresis with *Hae* III fragments of ∅X174 RF DNA as standards (Huang et al., 1973). The sizing of these ∅X174 fragments was subsequently found to be erroneous and, therefore, so are our previously published estimates for the SV40 fragments. A revised estimate of *Hae* III fragment sizes has been made by analyzing the relative amount of radioactivity in each limit fragment after digestion of [^{32}P] uniformly labeled SV40 DNA by *Hae* III and subsequent resolution of the 10 fragments on long (60 cm) cylindrical acrylamide gels.

> Revised estimates for the Pagano large plaque virus strain are:
> *Hae* III-A, 32.9 percent (1,630 base pairs);
> *Hae* III-B, 14.0 percent (690 base pairs);
> *Hae* III-C, 11.1 percent (550 base pairs);
> *Hae* III-D, 8.7 percent (430 base pairs);
> *Hae* III-E₁, 7.5 percent (370 base pairs);
> *Hae* III-E₂, 7.4 percent (365 base pairs);
> *Hae* III-F₁, 5.8 percent (287 base pairs);
> *Hae* III-F₂, 5.5 percent (273 base pairs);
> *Hae* III-G, 4.0 percent (200 base pairs); and
> *Hae* III-H, 3.1 percent (155 base pairs).

The *Hae* III-X fragment is estimated to be 220 base pairs. The transition from *Hae* III-E₂ to *Hae* III-F₁ involves a net deletion of about 80 base pairs; that from *Hae* III-F₁ to *Hae* III-X, about 65 base pairs.

Several different strategies are available for determining the unique order of the limit DNA fragments:

1. To isolate partial digestion products and redigest them to completion, thus identifying overlapping clusters of limit fragments;

2. To digest sequentially with two distinct restriction enzymes;

3. To use limit fragments as specific primers for the *in vitro* DNA repair synthesis of single-stranded template (SV40) DNA using the *E. coli* DNA polymerase I enzyme (Dumas, et al., 1971) and to determine by DNA-DNA hybridization which limit fragments are located adjacent to the specific primer; and

4. To isolate two distinct sets of limit fragments (using two distinct restriction enzymes) and to test by DNA-DNA hybridization all possible combinations of the two sets of limit fragments in order to monitor for possible overlaps.

Danna, Sack, and Nathans (1973) used a combination of strategies No. 1 and No. 2 to develop their cleavage map of SV40 DNA. Strategy No. 3 has been used by S. Summers (unpub. data) to order the *Hae* III fragments of polyoma DNA. Strategy No. 4 has been used in the analysis of the øX174 RF fragments (C. A. Hutchison, unpub.).

The ordering of the *Hae* III fragments remains incomplete, but some data has been obtained using strategy No. 1, the analysis of partial digestion products. Partial digestion products with the following limit fragment composition have been characterized: BC, CD, BCD, AD. This suggests the order BCDA and represents two-thirds of the genome. The precise order of the remaining six small limit fragments is still unknown. This partial ordering of the *Hae* III fragments can, however, be compared to the complete cleavage map of Danna, Sack, and Nathans (1973). The arbitrarily chosen origin for the SV40 mapping studies is the single unique cleavage site for the *Eco*RI restriction enzyme (Morrow and Berg, 1972; Mulder and Delius, 1972). In collaboration with E.-S. Huang and C. Mulder, the *Eco*RI site has been located in *Hae* III-B by a double digestion analysis; the *Hae* III-B fragment is cleaved by *Eco*RI into two subfragments of size 9.7 percent and 4.3 percent, respectively. However, which of the two possible locations of the *Eco*RI site with respect to the *Hae* III cleavage site which separates *Hae* III-B from *Hae* III-C cannot at present be deduced. Figure 2 displays the complete cleavage maps for the *Hind* (Fig. 2a) and *Hpa* (Figs. 2b and 2c) enzymes and the two possible representations of the *Hae* III cleavage sites (Figs. 2d and 2e) as presently mapped. The map shown in Figure 2d is currently favored since S. Weissman (pers. comm.) has mapped a promoter site for the *E. coli* DNA-dependent RNA polymerase at .16 map units. The promoter site is in the *Hind*-G fragment and is located internally within the *Hae* III-C fragment.

It has been mentioned that a physical cleavage map for the SV40 genome could serve as a reference for mapping other functions and properties of the viral chromosome. Information of this type has been compiled using the completed map of Danna, Sack, and Nathans (1973). The sites of origin and termination, and the direction of SV40 DNA replication have been determined (Danna and Nathans, 1972). Those portions of the SV40 DNA genome incorporated into the various adeno-SV40 hybrid viruses have been mapped (Morrow et al., 1973). Additionally, limit fragments have been identified as

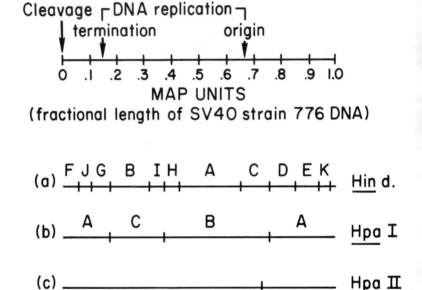

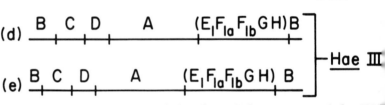

Figure 2. Linear representation of the physical cleavage map of the SV4
genome produced by the restriction endonucleases of *H. influenzae* (*Hind*)
H. parainfluenzae (*Hpa* I and *Hpa* II), and *H. aegyptius* (*Hae* III). The order
ing of the *Hae* III fragments remains incomplete: (d) and (e) are two alternat
possible arrangements.

representing "early" or "late" portions of the genome by hybridiza
tion with suitable probe RNAs (Huang et al., 1973; Khoury et al
1973; Sambrook et al., 1973).

My interest in the physical cleavage map and in an array c
specific DNA fragments was (1) to probe the relationship betwee
two prominent viral RNA species found in the cytoplasm of produc
tively infected cells and (2) to develop an *in vivo* transcription ma
for the SV40 genome. Earlier studies in collaboration with Z. Ber
Ishai and R. A. Weinberg demonstrated the presence of three di

tinct classes of viral RNA in the cytoplasm of monkey cells productively infected with SV40 (Weinberg et al., 1972). These viral RNA species have been designated the "early" 19S, "late" 19S, and "late" 16S according to the time of their appearance during lytic infection and their apparent size as judged by sedimentation on sucrose gradients. In addition, several independent cell lines transformed by SV40 have been shown to carry a prominent species of cytoplasmic viral RNA of about 19S (Weinberg et al., 1972, 1974). Many laboratories have demonstrated a high degree of sequence homology common to early lytic RNA and the viral RNA synthesized in SV40 transformed cells (Oda and Dulbecco, 1968; Aloni et al., 1968). Our evidence has not demonstrated absolute identity of molecular weight or nucleotide sequence for the early lytic and transformed viral transcripts. On the basis of the similar size of these two transcripts, however, we suggest that the 19S viral RNA species found in several SV40-transformed cell lines is related to the maintenance of the transformed state in such cells (Weinberg et al., 1974).

The bulk of the viral RNA late in the lytic cycle is apparently uniquely late RNA, i.e., viral RNA sequences whose transcription begins with the initiation of viral DNA replication. Only a minority of the viral RNA present late in the lytic cycle derives from continued transcription of early RNA (Weinberg et al., 1974). The uniquely late RNA consists of two size classes of RNA (Figure 3). The small late RNA (16S) is slightly smaller than 18S rRNA, whereas the large late RNA (19S) migrates in acrylamide gels at a position intermediate between 18S and 28S rRNAs. Figure 3a reveals the absence of any stable viral transcripts smaller than the 16S message. The profile of the late viral RNAs (Fig. 3) is found by using relatively long labeling periods. Briefer labeling periods show a preferential incorporation into the 19S species. Experiments employing brief pulse-labeling times, followed by a chase in the presence of actinomycin D (to block any further synthesis of viral RNA) clearly demonstrate that the 19S late RNA is metabolically less stable than the 16S late RNA (Weinberg et al., 1974). The general conclusion from these experiments is that the 16S late RNA is derived from the 19S late RNA by a mechanism occurring after these viral RNAs reach the cytoplasm of the infected cell (Weinberg et al., 1974). The suggested precursor-product relationship for the 19S and 16S late viral RNAs was not proven, however, since the pulse-chase experiments were unable to demonstrate unambiguously the transfer of labeled

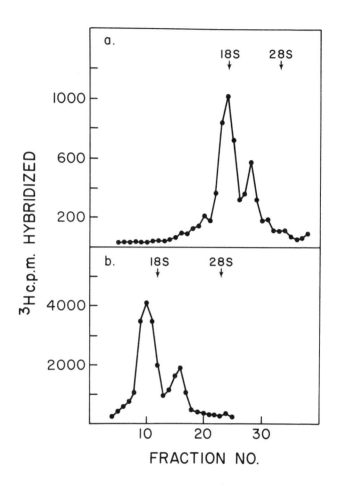

Figure 3.   Late SV40 specific RNA isolated from the cytoplasm of monkey kidney cells infected with the Vogt-Dulbecco strain of SV40 and fractionated by electrophoresis on 2.9 percent acrylamide gels. The viral RNA is extracted from infected cells labeled with [³H]uridine for 60 to 72 hours following infection, and is detected in the gel fractions by hybridization to nitrocellulose membrane filters loaded with 2 μg denatured SV40 DNA.

Figure 3a: electrophoresis is undertaken for 10 hours; hybridization is for 20 hours at 65 C in 2 x SSC followed by RNase treatment. Figure 3b: electrophoresis is for 20 hours; hybridization is for 30 hours at 37 C in 50 percent formamide and 1.0 M NaCl, and no RNase treatment. The positions of 18S and 28S rRNA species from the host cell are indicated by the arrows.

RNA from the 19S to the 16S species. The interpretation of the pulse-chase results was complicated by the observation that label was clearly being removed from both late RNA species during the chase, albeit more rapidly from the 19S than from the 16S (Weinberg et al., 1974).

Hybridization of these late viral RNA species to specific fragments of viral DNA offered an investigation of the sequence composition of these two transcripts. 19S and 16S late viral RNA preparations were made by pooling the appropriate fractions from an acrylamide gel similar to those shown in Figure 3. Each was then tested by DNA-RNA hybridization to the larger *Hae* III fragments of the Vogt-Dulbecco viral DNA (Table 2). Fragments *Hae* III-X, G, and H were not tested. The results demonstrate clearly that the 19S and 16S late viral species share nucleotide sequences. The data do not, however, clearly identify the existence of a set of sequences present in the 19S transcript not also present in the 16S species. Possibly the Hae III-E_1 fragment may prove to be such a sequence. The suggested approximate fragment compositions for the two late RNAs are as follows:

19S *Hae* III-B, C, E_1, F_{1a}, F_2
16S *Hae* III-B, C, F_{1a}, F_2

with fragments *Hae*-X, G, and H not yet analyzed. Other studies indicate fragments *Hae* III-A and D are early regions of the genome (Huang et al., 1973; Weinberg et al., 1974).

Table 2.   Hybridization of late SV40 messengers to *Hae* III fragments

Hae III fragment	16S RNA (Hybridized cpm)	19S RNA (Hybridized cpm)
A	8	6
B	532	436
C	274	230
D	9	8
E_1	35	108
$F_{1a} + F_2$	168	190

Note: In this experiment both mRNA and *Hae* III fragments were obtained using the Vogt-Dulbecco strain of SV40. The hybridization analysis is carried out using equi-molar amounts of the *Hae* III fragment DNA, immobilized onto nitrocellulose membrane filters, and hybridized under conditions of excess DNA.

The fragment compositions of the two late viral RNAs are compatible with the 19S being a precursor molecule to the 16S transcript. This type of data, however, does not constitute proof of such a precursor-product relationship. The fragment compositions are compatible with both the 16S and 19S species being derived from a distinct or a common nuclear precursor. The only compelling proof is an interpretable pulse-chase experiment, which so far has evaded us. The high degree of sequence identity exhibited by the two late viral RNAs in these experiments is in sharp contrast to the RNase T_1 fingerprint studies recently reported (Warnaar and deMol, 1973).

If one will accept the thesis that the 19S late RNA is a precursor of the 16S late transcript, then one can develop a cogent argument to infer the orientation of transcription of the late viral messages. Since both 16S and 19S late RNAs contain poly A sequences which first become associated with SV40 RNA in the nucleus of the infected cell (Weinberg et al., 1972), it seems reasonable to assume that the poly A sequences are conserved in the cytoplasmic processing of the 19S molecule into the 16S transcript. The poly A sequences are assumed to be located at the 3' end of the SV40 messages as demonstrated for other mammalian mRNAs (Greenberg and Perry, 1972). The simplest scheme for processing the 19S viral RNA in the cytoplasm and conserving the integrity of the 3' end of the molecule would therefore be by degradation from the 5' end (Fig. 4). Taken together with the partial fragment order given for the *Hae* III fragments in Figure 2, this would mean that the synthesis of the late viral messages would take place in the direction *Hae* III-E_1 through *Hae* III-B and into *Hae* III-C. Since it is known that early transcription uses one particular strand of the duplex genome as template while late transcription occurs on the other, it follows that the synthesis of early SV40 RNA takes place in the direction *Hae* III-A to *Hae* III-D. This inferred direction of SV40 transcription with respect to the cleavage map has been confirmed by more direct experiments (Khoury et al., 1973; Sambrook et al., 1973). The evidence previously discussed is presented in the form of a transcription map (Fig. 5). The precise locations for initiation and termination of synthesis for both early and late transcripts remain undefined. Moreover, the map displays the 19S and 16S late viral RNAs as being coterminous, which has not been definitely proven.

The analysis of the late SV40 messages raises the possibility that a particular late protein is translated from the 19S transcript and not

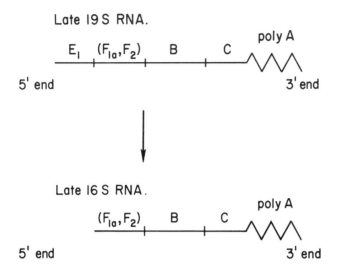

Note : <u>Hae</u> Ⅲ fragments – F_{Ib}, X, G or H have not been tested in this analysis.

Figure 4.   Schematic representation of the *Hae* III fragment composition of the two late viral RNA species.

from the 16S. The difference in molecular weight between the 16S and 19S RNA molecules is estimated to be 300,000 daltons, which is sufficient to encode a protein of 30,000 to 35,000 daltons. The minor capsid protein VP2 is estimated to be 32,000 daltons and would be expected to be made in a lower molar yield than VP1 (Estes et al., 1971). Presumably VP1, the major capsid protein (43,000 daltons), is translated from both 16S and 19S late viral RNAs. Thus, this scheme of late viral RNA metabolism may prove to be a means of regulating the molar yield of the different late proteins.

An unresolved problem emerging from these studies concerns the interpretation of the observed size of the early 19S viral message. The late 19S message is estimated to be 900,000 daltons, and the early 19S, 950,000 daltons. Together these two RNA molecules would represent a full transcript for SV40 DNA of 3.6 by 10^6 daltons, which suggests an approximate division of the genome into a 50 percent early region and a 50 percent late region. However, several laboratories using different nucleic acid hybridization techniques have esti-

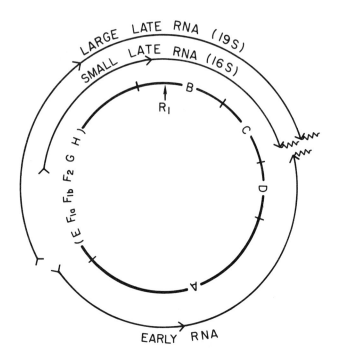

Figure 5.   Transcription map of SV40 strain 776. This map brings together the data of Table 2 and the schematic representation of Figure 4 with *Hae* III cleavage map of Figure 2d. The arrows indicate the direction of synthesis of transcription (from 5′ to 3′) for the stable viral RNA species. The polyA tails are indicated by the jagged line at the 3′ end of the RNA molecules.

mated the early region to be only 30 to 35 percent of the genome and the remaining 65 to 70 percent to be the late region (Oda and Dulbecco, 1968; Aloni et al., 1968; Lindstrom and Dulbecco, 1972; Khoury et al., 1972; Sambrook et al., 1972). The observed mass of the early 19S transcript is clearly larger than the transcript from the 30 to 35 percent of the genome allotted to the early functions. This apparent paradox in the present data would appear to have one of two possible solutions:

1. The combination of the two distinct 19S viral messages represents the full transcript of the SV40 genome; the genome is approximately equal in early and late functions. According to this interpretation, the experiments which fractionate the genome into a 30 to 35

percent early portion and a 65 to 70 percent late portion would have to be considered erroneous.

2. The early 19S viral RNA molecule represents a full transcript of that 35 percent of the genome which represents the early functions—about 600,000 daltons of RNA covalently attached to some 350,000 daltons of nonviral RNA sequences. Hybrid RNA molecules of mixed viral-cell sequences have, in fact, been reported in the SV40 lytic infection (Rozenblatt and Winocour, 1972), but such hybrid molecules are confined largely to the nucleus.

In conclusion, analysis of the SV40 genome by restriction endonuclease cleavage demonstrates the usefulness of these enzymes in probing the organization and function of small genomes. A specific region of the SV40 chromosome is revealed by analysis with the *Hae* III-enzyme to be capable of major sequence variations, involving net insertions and deletions of as much as 140 base pairs. This region has not yet been mapped precisely but probably lies within that portion of the genome encoding late functions. Direct evidence for the transcription of this portion of the genome is also not yet available, but the observed mass of the late viral RNA transcripts suggest that it probably is transcribed. Further analysis may possibly reveal this variable region of the genome to be an intergenic spacer region which is transcribed but not translated; possibly it will be found in the late 19S transcript but not in the late 16S. These questions remain for future experiments.

Looking ahead, it is clear that these restriction enzymes will be useful for the analysis of integrated viral genomes in cells transformed by either DNA or RNA tumor viruses and, as our techniques improve, for probing the structure and function of the eukaryote chromosome itself.

Acknowledgments: The author is extremely grateful to D. Nathans for making available his data on the *Hin*d and *Hpa* cleavages prior to their publication. This work was supported in part by grant 5RO1-CA-14572-02 from the National Cancer Institute.

Addendum in proof: P. Lebowitz, W. Siefel, and J. Sklar (pers. comm.) have recently derived a complete map of the *Hae* III fragments of SV40 DNA which confirms the mapping reported here. Furthermore these workers, and independently W. Fiers, have shown that the *Hae* III enzyme generates six to eight very small (20-40 base pairs) specific limit fragments in addition to the ten major fragments of SV40 DNA described in this paper.

Literature Cited

Aloni, Y., E. Winocour, and L. Sachs. 1968. Characterization of the simian virus 40-specific RNA in virus-yielding and transformed cells. J. Mol. Biol., *31:* 415-429.

Danna, K. J., and D. Nathans. 1972. Bidirectional replication of simian virus 40 DNA. Proc. Nat. Acad. Sci. U.S., *69:* 3097-3100.

Danna, K. J., G. H. Sack, Jr., and D. Nathans. 1973. Studies of simian virus 40 DNA. VII. A cleavage map of the SV40 genome. J. Mol. Biol., *78:* 363-376.

Dumas, L. B., G. Darby, and R. L. Sinsheimer. 1971. The replication of bacteriophage øX174 DNA *in vitro.* Temperature effects on repair synthesis and displacement synthesis. Biochim. Biophys. Acta, *228:* 407-422.

Estes, M. K., E.-S. Huang, and J. S. Pagano. 1971. Structural polypeptides of simian virus 40. J. Virol., *7:* 635-641.

Greenberg, J. R., and R. P. Perry. 1972. Isolation and characterization of steady state labeled messenger RNA from L-cells. Biochim. Biophys. Acta, *287:* 361-366.

Huang, E.-S., J. E. Newbold, and J. S. Pagano. 1973. Analysis of simian virus 40 DNA with the restriction enzyme of *Haemophilus aegyptius,* endonuclease Z. J. Virol., *11:* 508-514.

Khoury, G., J. C. Byrne, and M. A. Martin. 1972. Patterns of simian virus 40 DNA transcription after acute infection of permissive and nonpermissive cells. Proc. Nat. Acad. Sci. U.S., *69:* 1925-1928.

Khoury, G., M. A. Martin, T. N. H. Lee, K. J. Danna, and D. Nathans. 1973. A map of simian virus 40 transcription sites expressed in productively infected cells. J. Mol. Biol., *78:* 377-389.

Lindstrom, D. M., and R. Dulbecco. 1972. Strand orientation of simian virus 40 transcription in productively infected cells. Proc. Nat. Acad. Sci. U.S., *69:* 1517-1520.

Morrow, J. F., and P. Berg. 1972. Cleavage of simian virus 40 DNA at a unique site by a bacterial restriction enzyme. Proc. Nat. Acad. Sci. U.S., *69:* 3365-3369.

Morrow, J. F., P. Berg, T. J. Kelly, Jr., and A. M. Lewis, Jr. 1973. Mapping of simian virus 40 early functions on the viral chromosome. J. Virol., *12:* 653-658.

Mulder, C., and H. Delius. 1972. Specificity of the break produced by restricting endonuclease R, in simian virus 40 DNA, as revealed by partial denaturation mapping. Proc. Nat. Acad. Sci. U.S., *69:* 3215-3219.

Oda, K., and R. Dulbecco. 1968. Regulation of transcription of the SV40 DNA in productively infected and in transformed cells. Proc. Nat. Acad. Sci. U.S., *60:* 525-532.

Rozenblatt, S., and E. Winocour. 1972. Covalently linked cell and SV40 specific sequences in an RNA from productively infected cells. Virology, *50:* 558-566.

Sambrook, J., P. A. Sharp, and W. Keller. 1972. Transcription of simian virus 40 DNA and hybridization of the separated strands to RNA extracted from lytically infected and transformed cells. J. Mol. Biol., *70:* 57-71.

Sambrook, J., B. Sugden, W. Keller, and P. A. Sharp. 1973. Transcription of simian virus. III. Mapping of "early" and "late" species of RNA. Proc. Nat. Acad. Sci. U.S., *70:* 3711-3715.

Smith, H. O., and D. Nathans. 1973. A suggested nomenclature for bacterial host modification and restriction systems and their enzymes. J. Mol. Biol., *81:* 419-423.

Warnaar, S. O., and A. W. de Mol. 1973. Characterization of two simian virus 40-specific RNA molecules from infected BS-C-1 cells. J. Virol., *12:* 124-129.

Weinberg, R. A., Z. Ben-Ishai, and J. E. Newbold. 1972. Poly A associated with SV40 messenger RNA. Nature New Biol., *238:* 111-113.

Weinberg, R. A., Z. Ben-Ishai, and J. E. Newbold. 1974. Simian virus 40 transcription in productively infected and transformed cells. J. Virol., *13:* 1263-1273.

The Structure and Replication of the Adenovirus Genome

GEORGE D. PEARSON
Department of Biochemistry and Biophysics
Oregon State University
Corvallis, Oregon

IN RECENT YEARS, adenoviruses have received increasing attention as a model system to study viral oncogenesis. This is due in part to the development of detailed genetic and physical maps, the identification of specific regions of the adenovirus chromosome in transformed cell lines, the transformation of cells with defined fragments of adenovirus DNA, the mapping of messenger RNA molecules, and the extensive information about structural and nonstructural viral polypeptides (see, for example, Cold Spring Harbor Symp. Quant. Biol., 39, 1974. In spite of this explosive progress, the mechanism of adenovirus replication remains open to question. This paper reviews the DNA structure and replication of the closely related type 2 and type 5 adenoviruses.

THE ADENOVIRUS CHROMOSOME

The linear adenovirus chromosome has a molecular weight of 23×10^6. The sequence of the chromosome, determined by denaturation mapping (Doerfler and Kleinschmidt, 1970), is not circularly permuted. The AT-rich half of the molecule has been defined as the right end. After shearing, the halves can be separated in $Hg(II)$-Cs_2SO_4 density gradients (Kimes and Green, 1970; Doerfler and Kleinschmidt, 1970). Site-specific endonucleases cleave adenovirus DNA into unique fragments (Pettersson et al., 1973; Sharp et al., 1973; Mulder et al., 1974a). Figure 1 shows the sizes and order of

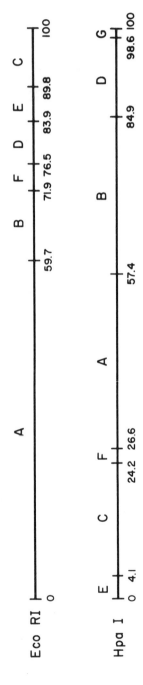

Figure 1. Physical order of type 2 adenovirus DNA fragments generated by cleavage with *Eco*RI and *Hpa* I restriction endonucleases. The scale is percent of genome molecular weight.

fragments generated by restriction endonucleases *Eco*RI, isolated from *Escherichia coli* harboring an fi⁺ resistance transfer factor, and *Hpa* I, isolated from *Haemophilus parainfluenzae*. The *Eco*RI-A fragment includes the GC-rich, or left, end of the chromosome (Mulder et al., 1974b).

The intact strands can be separated in CsCl density gradients after complexing with poly IG (Kubinski and Rose, 1967) or poly UG (Landgraf-Leurs and Green, 1971). They also separate in alkaline CsCl density gradients (Sussenbach et al., 1973). The strand that bands at the lower density in poly UG gradients corresponds to the dense strand in alkaline CsCl gradients (Tibbetts et al., 1974). Sharp and co-workers (1974) recently showed that the 3′ terminus of the heavy alkaline strand lies to the left on the physical map in fragment *Hpa* I-E. The 3′ terminus of the light alkaline strand is in *Hpa* I-G. This information completely defines the topography of the chromosome.

REPLICATING ADENOVIRUS CHROMOSOMES

Synchronized cells infected at the beginning of S-phase proceed normally through S-phase, but do not enter mitosis nor initiate a subsequent round of cellular DNA synthesis (Hodge and Scharff, 1969; Pearson and Hanawalt, 1971; Simmons et al., 1974). Since viral replication begins after cellular replication has ceased, adenovirus DNA can be labeled exclusively.

Adenoviruses replicate in the nuclei of infected cells. Viral DNA most likely exists within the nucleus as a nucleoprotein complex. Pearson and Hanawalt (1971) isolated nascent viral DNA in the form of a replication complex. The kinetics of labeling established that the adenovirus complex was an intermediate in replication. Studies with three complementation groups of type 31 adenovirus temperature-sensitive mutants, all defective in the initiation of viral DNA synthesis, showed that the replication complex does not form at nonpermissive temperatures (Shiroki and Shimojo, 1974; Suzuki and Shimojo, 1974). The complex contains two virus-specified DNA binding proteins as well as endonuclease and DNA polymerase activities (Yamashita and Green, 1974; Yamashita, Arens, and Green, pers. comm.). Electron microscope autoradiography indicates that viral DNA synthesis occurs in the nucleoplasm, not in association with the nuclear envelope (Shiroki et al., 1974; Simmons et al., 1974).

Therefore, the intranuclear site of replication has not yet been identified.

Nascent viral DNA, extracted either from the replication complex (Pearson and Hanawalt, 1971; Pearson, 1975) or directly from cells (Sussenbach et al., 1972; Bellett and Younghusband, 1972; van der Eb, 1973; Pettersson, 1973), differs physically from mature molecules. For example, replicating DNA has an increased buoyant density and a greater sedimentation coefficient. Figure 2A shows that after labeling viral DNA for 15 minutes, two peaks at densities of 1.605 and 1.585 appeared in a CsCl gradient containing ethidium bromide. Shorter pulses predominantly labeled the dense band. A

Figure 2.   Characterization of replicating and completed adenovirus DNA. Synchronized, infected cells were concentrated to 1.7 x 10⁶ cells/ml and labeled for 15 minutes with [³H]thymidine (10 μCi/ml at 6.7 Ci/nmole). DNA was extracted from whole cells with chloroform-isoamyl alcohol after digestion with 1 mg pronase/ml and 2 percent sodium dodecyl sulfate.

Panel A: Equilibrium centrifugation of extracted DNA in a CsCl density gradient (initial ρ = 1.550) containing 300 μg ethidium bromide/ml. Fractions labeled b and c were pooled separately, extracted with isopropanol, and dialyzed. [¹⁴C]-HeLa DNA (not shown) co-banded with the light band (c). The density increases from right to left.

Panel B: Rebanding of fraction b and [¹⁴C]-HeLa DNA (not shown) in a neutral CsCl density gradient (initial ρ = 1.710). Fractions labeled e were pooled and dialyzed. The vertical dashed lines represent, from left to right: replicating viral DNA, adenovirus DNA, and HeLa DNA.

Panel C: Rebanding of fraction c and [¹⁴C]-HeLa (not shown) in a neutral CsCl density gradient. Fractions labeled f were pooled and dialyzed.

Panel D: Rebanding of a mixture of b and c in a neutral CsCl density gradient. Closed circles represent marker [¹⁴C]-HeLa DNA.

Panel E: Neutral sucrose gradient velocity sedimentation of fraction e. Sucrose gradients (containing 1.0 M NaCl, 0.005 M EDTA, and 0.01 M Tris, pH 8) were centrifuged for 7 hours at 25,000 rpm. Fractions labeled h and i were pooled separately and dialyzed. Sedimentation is from right to left.

Panel F: Neutral sucrose gradient velocity sedimentation of fraction f. The fraction labeled j was retained and dialyzed.

Panel G: Neutral sucrose gradient velocity sedimentation of a mixture of e and f. The arrow marks the position of 42S.

Panel H: Rebanding of fraction h in a neutral CsCl density gradient. ●————●, [¹⁴C]-HeLa DNA. The vertical dashed lines represent, from left to right: replicating viral DNA, adenovirus DNA, and HeLa DNA.

Panel I: Rebanding of fraction i and [¹⁴C]-HeLa DNA (not shown) in a neutral CsCl density gradient.

Panel J: Rebanding of fraction j and [¹⁴C]-HeLa DNA (not shown) in a neutral CsCl density gradient.

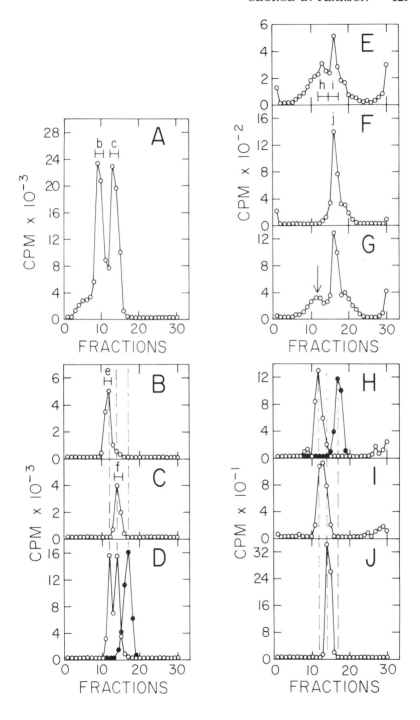

subsequent chase with unlabeled thymidine transferred label in the dense peak to the light peak. These kinetic experiments confirm a precursor-product relationship. When centrifuged in CsCl gradients after removing the ethidium bromide, the dense peak banded at a density of 1.725 (Fig. 2B) and the light peak banded at 1.715 (Fig. 2C), the density of mature adenovirus DNA. Figure 2D shows that two peaks with the expected densities appeared when both bands were mixed. No pulse label was found in the region of cellular DNA in the CsCl gradients. Figure 2E demonstrates that replicating DNA, isolated as the dense CsCl band, sedimented at 31S or greater. Some of the molecules sedimented as fast as 60S. The light CsCl band sedimented at 31S (Fig. 2F), the rate for mature viral DNA. No molecules sedimented faster than 31S. When a mixture of both dense and light bands was centrifuged, a fast-sedimenting peak appeared in addition to the 31S peak (Fig. 2G). Replicating DNA sedimenting between 35S and 40S (fractions marked h in Fig. 2E) banded at a density of 1.725 as shown in Figure 2H. Replicating DNA sedimenting near 31S (fractions labeled i in Fig. 2E) banded at a slightly lower density, spanning the region between 1.715 and 1.725. Mature 31S DNA, previously isolated at a density of 1.715, remained at the same density (Fig. 2J).

Nascent viral strands longer than unit length never have been demonstrated (Horwitz, 1971). When labeled for one minute or less, replicating molecules contain 10S chains (Pearson, 1975), corresponding to about 1/20 of a unit strand. Vlak and co-workers (1975) and Winnacker (1975) have shown that 9S to 11S nascent strands are complementary to both viral strands throughout the entire genome. Since these short chains can be chased into full-length strands, adenoviruses replicate discontinuously. The average time required for adenovirus replication is 16 to 17 minutes, a rate of 0.7 x 10^6 daltons per minute for chain elongation (Pearson, 1975). Although newly finished molecules sediment at 31S and have a density of 1.715, they still contain single-stranded interruptions (Pearson, 1975). Mature chromosomes do not. Complete joining of daughter strands requires at least an additional 15 to 20 minutes (Pearson, unpub.). Unjoined strands are approximately 0.25, 0.5, and 0.75 fractional lengths. The significance of this observation will be discussed below.

Since treatment with single-strand specific endonucleases, but not with ribonuclease, lowers the buoyant density of replicating viral

DNA without the loss of the pulse label, a substantial fraction of the *parental* strands must be single-stranded (Pettersson, 1973; Pearson, 1975). Branched and unbranched linear molecules containing extensive single-stranded regions have been visualized in the electron microscope (Sussenbach et al., 1972; van der Eb, 1973). The DNA molecules can be classified into three groups: single strands of unit length or less, branched molecules containing either one single-stranded arm or one partially single-stranded arm, and unit length unbranched molecules containing single-stranded regions. The displaced strand corresponds to the heavy alkaline strand (Sussenbach and van der Vliet, 1973). By denaturation mapping, Ellens and coworkers (1974) identified the *unreplicated* portion of the branched molecules as the GC-rich, or left, end of the chromosome. No evidence was found for circular or concatemeric replicative intermediates. Robinson and co-workers (1973) recently extracted from virus particles a DNA-protein complex which subsequently circularizes. Only linear molecules were recovered after deproteinization. This may explain why only linear-replicating molecules have been seen in the electron microscope.

ADENOVIRUS REPLICATION MAP

Danna and Nathans (1972) pioneered a method to map the origin and direction of replication of SV40 DNA. Infected cells are exposed to a short pulse of radioactivity during viral replication. Finished molecules, separated from replicating molecules, are cleaved with a site-specific endonuclease. The most heavily labeled fragments define the terminus of replication. Conversely, fragments from the region of the chromosome synthesized first will contain the least amount of label. This strategy, which requires no assumptions about the *structure* of replicating molecules, has also been used to determine the replication order of polyoma DNA (Crawford et al., 1974) and ϕX174 DNA (Godson, 1974).

Pearson (1976) constructed a replication map of adenovirus using the *Eco*RI restriction endonuclease. Figure 3 illustrates the purification of *Eco*RI adenovirus fragments by electrophoresis in a 0.7 percent agarose gel. The physical order of the fragments is compared in Figure 4 with the relative specific activity of each fragment from pulse-labeled, newly completed molecules. After a 5-minute pulse, a gradient of labeling increases from fragment F towards frag-

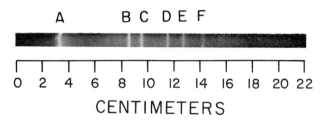

Figure 3. Preparative agarose gel electrophoresis of *Eco*RI fragments of type 2 adenovirus DNA. The gel contains about 50 μg of cleaved DNA. Electrophoresis on 0.7 percent agarose gels (1.2 cm x 30 cm) was for 7 hours at 20 ma. After staining with 0.5 μg ethidium bromide/ml, the fragment bands were visualized with long-wave ultraviolet light. The anode is to the right.

ment C, the right molecular end. The gradient of labeling disappears with pulse times longer than 15 to 20 minutes. An origin is located internally either in fragment F or in fragment B very near to F. Fragments B and C contain replicative termini. Three additional termini within fragment A can be estimated from the quantitative labeling data. Winnacker (1974) has evidence for at least another origin in *Eco*RI-A, in the region defined by the *Hpa* I-F fragment (see Fig. 1). Thus, two replicative origins are positioned about 25 percent from either end of the chromosome. Horwitz (1974) also has demonstrated origins in both halves of the adenovirus genome using a similar procedure. During recovery from hydroxyurea, when synthesis on the displaced strand is inhibited (Sussenbach and van der Vliet, 1973), a single origin at the right end can be detected (Ellens et al., 1974).

A tentative interpretation of adenovirus replication based on these data is diagrammed in Figure 5. The light alkaline strand (Sussenbach et al., 1973) is used as a template for leftward replication starting in fragment C and ending in fragment A. The heavy alkaline parental strand is displaced. A similar mechanism has been proposed for mitochondrial DNA replication (Robberson and Clayton, 1972, 1973; Berk and Clayton, 1974). There are four origins for rightward synthesis on the displaced strand: one at the left end, one about 25 percent from the left end (in *Hpa* I-F), one near the middle of the chromosome, and one in *Eco*RI-F. These distances roughly correspond to the sizes of unjoined daughter strands present in newly finished molecules (see discussion above). Unbranched molecules with several single-stranded gaps have been visualized by electron microscopy (Sussenbach et al., 1972; van der Eb, 1973; Ellens et al., 1974).

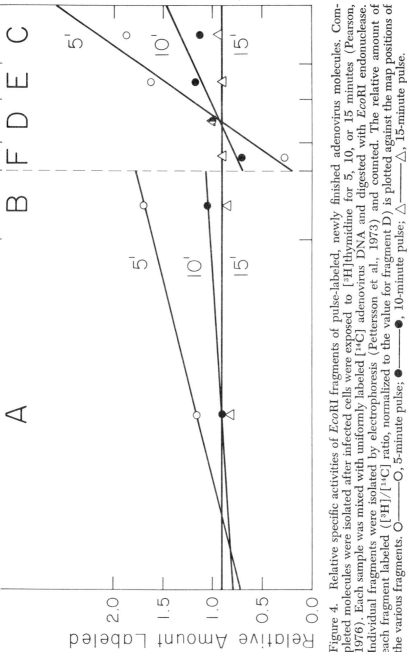

Figure 4. Relative specific activities of EcoRI fragments of pulse-labeled, newly finished adenovirus molecules. Completed molecules were exposed after infected cells were exposed to [³H]thymidine for 5, 10, or 15 minutes (Pearson, 1976). Each sample was mixed with uniformly labeled [¹⁴C] adenovirus DNA and digested with EcoRI endonuclease. Individual fragments were isolated by electrophoresis (Pettersson et al., 1973) and counted. The relative amount of each fragment labeled ([³H]/[¹⁴C] ratio, normalized to the value for fragment D) is plotted against the map positions of the various fragments. O———O, 5-minute pulse; ●———●, 10-minute pulse; △———△, 15-minute pulse.

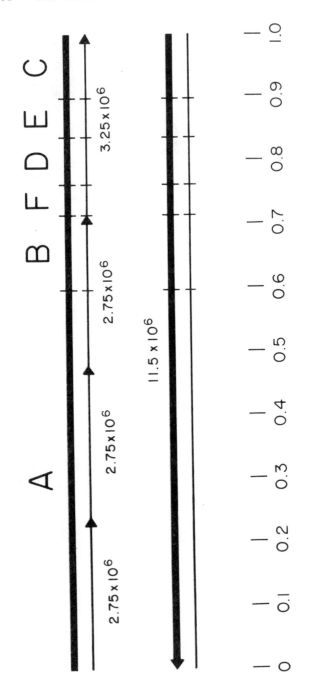

Figure 5. The positions of origins and termini of replication on adenovirus DNA. The upper diagram shows rightward replication using the heavy alkaline strand (thick line) as a template. The termini are indicated by the arrowheads. The arrows point in the 5′ to 3′ direction. Leftward replication using the light alkaline strand (thin line) is illustrated in the lower diagram. The terminus of replication is again indicated by the arrowhead. The letters represent EcoRI fragments. The scale is fraction of molecular length.

t is tempting to speculate that unjoined strands are sealed at the junctions between origins and termini. The polarity and orientation of the strands are correct (Sharp et al., 1974). This model predicts that during recovery from hydroxyurea inhibition, a single terminus located in *Eco*RI-A should be labeled. The gradient of labeling should *decrease* from left to right (ABFDEC). A further prediction is that only the light alkaline strand in *Eco*RI-C should be labeled during a short pulse.

THE ADENOVIRUS TERMINAL REPETITION

Watson (1972) has argued that linear molecules must have terminally repetitious sequences in order to form circular or concatemeric intermediates during replication. The replication of a linear chromosome is diagrammed in Figure 6. Only one of the template strands (a) is shown for simplicity. The primer, shown as small circles in (b), can be a short stretch of RNA (Winnacker, 1975). The heavy line in (c) represents the complementary daughter strand. It grows in the 5′ to 3′ direction. If the primer is subsequently removed by ribonuclease H, the 3′ terminus of the template strand will project as a tail from the otherwise duplex rod (d). The missing segment cannot be completed since DNA polymerase cannot add deoxyribonucleotides to the 5′ terminus of the daughter strand. Now consider

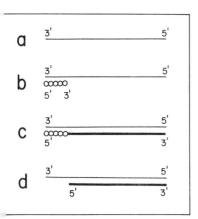
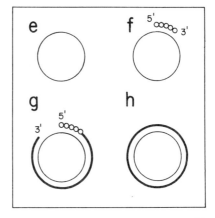

Figure 6.   DNA synthesis on a linear (*a* through *d*) or a circular (*e* through *h*) template. 3′ and 5′ refer respectively to the 3′-hydroxyl and 5′-phosphoryl termini. Thin line, template strand; thick line, newly synthesized DNA; small open circles, primer RNA.

the replication of a circular molecule. Again only a single template strand is shown (e). The primer (f) and the daughter strand (g) remain as described for the linear chromosome. After removal of the primer, continued DNA synthesis yields a nicked duplex circle which can be sealed by DNA ligase into a covalently closed circle (h). The daughter strand is complete.

The adenovirus molecule is not terminally repetitious in the usual sense (Greene et al., 1967). Figure 7 shows, however, that each strand can form hydrogen-bonded, single-stranded circles (Garon et al., 1972; Wolfson and Dressler, 1972). A simple conclusion is that the molecule has an *inverted* terminal repetition. Robert:

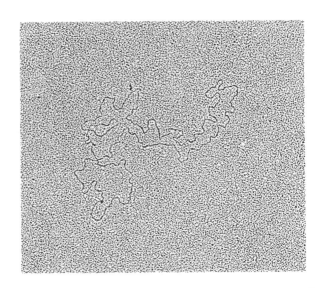

Figure 7.   Electron micrograph of a single-stranded adenovirus circle. The pro cedure of Garon, Berry, and Rose (1972) was used to form circles. Molecule were mounted for electron microscopy as described by Inman and Schne (1970). (Courtesy of David Coombs).

and co-workers (1974) estimate that the repetition is between 10 to 140 nucleotide pairs long.

Four general arrangements that could account for single stranded ring formation are illustrated in Figure 8. Structures (c and (d) are likely excluded since the circles are converted to linea strands after digestion with exonuclease III which removes mononu cleotides from the 3′ ends of duplex DNA. Of the remaining possibil

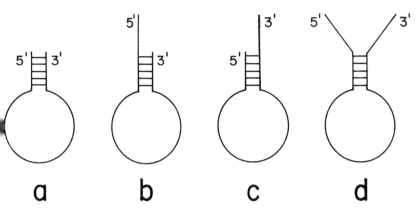

Figure 8.   Four general structures for adenovirus single-stranded circles. In each case, the two ends of either strand can form base pairs to form a region of double-stranded DNA. In (a) the ends of the strand are base paired out to the 3' and 5' termini. In (b) the region of base pairing ends before reaching the 5' terminus, leaving a single-stranded tail. In (c) the base pairing ends before reaching the 3' terminus, again leaving a tail. In (d) the termini are not base paired. (Adapted from Wolfson and Dressler, 1972).

ies, structure (b) is particularly interesting in light of the mechanism proposed for circularizing linear single-strands of ⌀X174 DNA Iwaya et al., 1973). Imagine that the phosphorylated 5' end can loop back near to the 3' end in a limited duplex region (Fig. 9, structure (a)). This structure is still a substrate for exonuclease III. Unless there is a gap, ligase can join the ends to form a covalently closed circular template (b). Otherwise, a combination of DNA polymerase and ligase can close a gap. After synthesis of the daughter strand (c), the replicated molecule contains a sequence with two-fold rotational symmetry (although not explicitly noted, there may be nicks or gaps in this molecule). The sequence can "loop out," perhaps in response to a specific polymeric protein, as shown in (d). This structure has been advanced as an intermediate in recombination pathways (Sobell, 1972). A double-stranded endonucleolytic attack yields the linear molecule (e). Replication by a strand displacement mechanism (Sussenbach and van der Vliet, 1973; Ellens et al., 1974) regenerates the free single strand (a). One of the striking features of the model outlined in Figure 9 is that the ends of the linear duplex molecule (e) fold back as hairpins. As a consequence, the nucleotide sequence at the 3' terminus of one strand is not necessarily complementary to the sequence at the 5' terminus of the other strand. Bate-

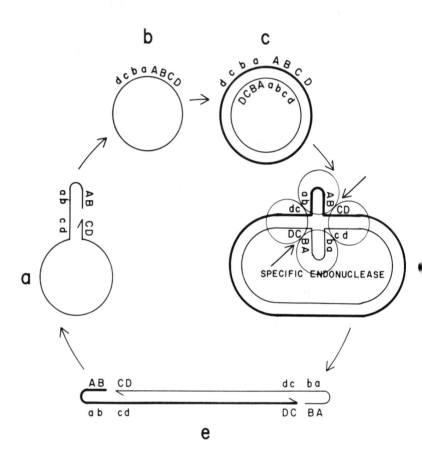

Figure 9.   Structure and role of the inverted terminal repetition in adenovir
DNA. Complementary sequences are indicated by upper and lower case lette
In (a) and (e) the 3'-hydroxyl terminus is specified by an arrowhead. T
arrows in (d) show the sites of endonucleolytic cleavage. The details of t
replication cycle are explained in the text.

man (1975) has developed an alternative model, modified from a
earlier proposal by Cavalier-Smith (1974), for the replication
linear molecules which involves hairpin ends. Experiments are
progress to test for the presence of hairpin regions in the adenovir
chromosome.

Acknowledgments: Research by the author was supported by grants (NP-67, NP-67A) from the American Cancer Society. Part of the work was done as a Dernham Junior Fellow (J-126) of the California Division of the American Cancer Society.

I thank Ron Davis, Herbert Boyer, and Lyle Brown for timely and generous gifts of *Eco*RI endonuclease. Gail Foster, Marda Brown, and Mark Engelking provided excellent technical assistance.

Literature Cited

Bateman, A. J. 1975. Simplification of palindromic telomere theory. Nature (London), *253:* 379.

Bellett, A. J. D., and H. B. Younghusband. 1972. Replication of the DNA of chick embryo lethal orphan virus. J. Mol. Biol., *72:* 691-709.

Berk, A. J., and D. A. Clayton. 1974. Mechanism of mitochondrial DNA replication in mouse L-cells; asynchronous replication of strands, segregation of circular daughter molecules, aspects of topology and turnover of an initiation sequence. J. Mol. Biol., *86:* 801-824.

Cavalier-Smith, T. 1974. Palindromic base sequences and replication of eukaryote chromosome ends. Nature (London), *250:* 467-470.

Crawford, L. V., A. K. Robbins, and P. M. Nicklin. 1974. Location of the origin and terminus of replication in polyoma virus DNA. J. Gen. Virol., *25:* 133-142.

Danna, K. J., and D. Nathans. 1972. Bidirectional replication of simian virus 40 DNA. Proc. Nat. Acad. Sci. U.S., *69:* 3097-3100.

Doerfler, W., and A. K. Kleinschmidt. 1970. Denaturation pattern of the DNA of adenovirus type 2 as determined by electron microscopy. J. Mol. Biol., *50:* 579-593.

Ellens, D. J., J. S. Sussenbach, and H. S. Jansz. 1974. Studies on the mechanism of replication of adenovirus DNA. III. Electron microscopy of replicating DNA. Virology, *61:* 427-442.

Garon, C. F., K. W. Berry, and J. A. Rose. 1972. A unique form of terminal redundancy in adenovirus DNA molecules. Proc. Nat. Acad. Sci. U.S., *69:* 2391-2395.

Godson, G. N. 1974. Origin and direction of ϕX174 double- and single-stranded DNA synthesis. J. Mol. Biol., *90:* 127-141.

Green, M., M. Piña, R. Kimes, P. C. Wensink, L. A. MacHattie, and C. A. Thomas Jr. 1967. Adenovirus DNA. I. Molecular weight and conformation. Proc. Nat. Acad. Sci. U.S., *57:* 1302-1309.

Hodge, L .D., and M. D. Scharff. 1969. Effect of adenovirus on host cell DNA synthesis in synchronized cells. Virology, *37:* 554-564.

Horwitz, M. S. 1971. Intermediates in the synthesis of type 2 adenovirus deoxyribonucleic acid. J. Virol., *8:* 675-683.

Horwitz, M. S. 1974. Location of the origin of DNA replication in adenovirus type 2. J. Virol., *13:* 1046-1054.

Inman, R. B., and M. Schnös. 1970. Partial denaturation of thymine- and 5-bromouracil-containing λDNA in alkali. J. Mol. Biol., 49: 93-98.

Iwaya, M., S. Eisenberg, K. Bartok, and D. T. Denhardt. 1973. Mechanism of replication of single-stranded ϕX174 DNA. VII. Circularization of the progeny viral strand. J. Virol., 12: 808-818.

Kimes, R., and M. Green. 1970. Adenovirus DNA. II. Separation of molecular halves of adenovirus type 2 DNA. J. Mol. Biol., 50: 203-206.

Kubinski, H., and J. A. Rose. 1967. Regions containing repeating base-pairs in DNA from some oncogenic and non-oncogenic animal viruses. Proc. Nat. Acad. Sci. U.S., 57: 1720-1725.

Landgraf-Leurs, M., and M. Green. 1971. Adenovirus DNA. III. Separation of the complementary strands of adenovirus 2, 7 and 12 DNA molecules. J. Mol. Biol., 60: 185-202.

Mulder, C., P. A. Sharp, H. Delius, and U. Pettersson. 1974a. Specific fragmentation of DNA of adenovirus serotypes 3, 5, 7, and 12, and adeno-simian virus 40 hybrid virus Ad 2+ NDl by restriction endonuclease R • EcoRI. J. Virol., 14: 68-77.

Mulder, C., J. R. Arrand, H. Delius, W. Keller, U. Pettersson, R. J. Roberts, and P. A. Sharp. 1974b. Cleavage maps of DNA from adenovirus types 2 and 5 by restriction endonucleases EcoRI and Hpa I. Cold Spring Harbor Symp. Quant. Biol., 39: 397-400.

Pearson, G. D. 1975. An intermediate in adenovirus type 2 replication. J. Virol., 16: 17-26.

Pearson, G. D. 1976. Replication map of type 2 adenovirus. Proc. Nat. Acad. Sci. U.S., 73:in press.

Pearson, G. D., and P. C. Hanawalt. 1971. Isolation of DNA replication complexes from uninfected and adenovirus-infected HeLa cells. J. Mol. Biol., 62: 65-80.

Pettersson, U. 1973. Some unusual properties of replicating adenovirus type 2 DNA. J. Mol. Biol., 81: 521-527.

Pettersson, U., C. Mulder, H. Delius, and P. Sharp. 1973. Cleavage of adenovirus type 2 DNA into six unique fragments by endonuclease R•RI. Proc. Nat. Acad. Sci. U.S., 70: 200-204.

Robberson, D. L., and D. A. Clayton. 1972. Replication of mitochondrial DNA in mouse L cells and their thymidine kinase derivatives: Displacement replication on a covalently-closed circular template. Proc. Nat. Acad. Sci. U.S., 69: 3810-3814.

Robberson, D. L., and D. A. Clayton. 1973. Pulse-labeled components in the replication of mitochondrial deoxyribonucleic acid. J. Biol. Chem., 248: 4512-4514.

Roberts, R. J., J. R. Arrand, and W. Keller. 1974. The length of the terminal repetition in adenovirus-2 DNA. Proc. Nat. Acad. Sci. U.S., 71: 3829-3833.

Robinson, A. J., H. B. Younghusband, and A. J. D. Bellett. 1973. A circular DNA-protein complex from adenoviruses. Virology, 56: 54-69.

Sharp, P. A., P. H. Gallimore, and S. J. Flint. 1974. Mapping of adenovirus 2 RNA sequences in lytically infected cells and transformed cell lines. Cold Spring Harbor Symp. Quant. Biol., 39: 457-474.

Sharp, P. A., B. Sugden, and J. Sambrook. 1973. Detection of two restriction endonuclease activities in *Haemophilus parainfluenzae* using analytical agarose-ethidium bromide electrophoresis. Biochemistry, *12:* 3055-3063.

Shiroki, K., and H. Shimojo. 1974. Analysis of adenovirus 12 temperature-sensitive mutants defective in viral DNA replication. Virology, *61:* 474-485.

Shiroki, K., H. Shimojo, and K. Yamaguchi. 1974. The viral DNA replication complex of adenovirus 12. Virology, *60:* 192-199.

Simmons, T., P. Heywood, and L. D. Hodge. 1974. Intranuclear site of replication of adenovirus DNA. J. Mol. Biol., *89:* 423-433.

Sobell, H. M. 1972. Molecular mechanism for genetic recombination. Proc. Nat. Acad. Sci. U.S., *69:* 2483-2487.

Sussenbach, J. S., and P. C. van der Vliet. 1973. Studies on the mechanism of replication of adenovirus DNA. I. The effect of hydroxyurea. Virology, *54:* 299-303.

Sussenbach, J. S., D. J. Ellens, and H. S. Jansz. 1973. Studies on the mechanism of replication of adenovirus DNA. J. Virol., *12:* 1131-1138.

Sussenbach, J. S., P. C. van der Vliet, D. J. Ellens, and H. S. Jansz. 1972. Linear intermediates in the replication of adenovirus DNA. Nature New Biol., *239:* 47-49.

Suzuki, E., and H. Shimojo. 1974. Temperature-sensitive formation of the DNA replication complex in adenovirus 31-infected cells. J. Virol., *13:* 538-540.

Tibbetts, C., U. Pettersson, K. Johansson, and L. Philipson. 1974. Relationship of mRNA from productively infected cells to the complementary strands of adenovirus type 2 DNA. J. Virol., 13: 370-377.

van der Eb, A. J. 1973. Intermediates in type 5 adenovirus DNA replication. Virology, *51:* 11-23.

Vlak, J. M., Th. H. Rozijn, and J. S. Sussenbach. 1975. Studies on the mechanism of replication of adenovirus DNA. IV. Discontinuous DNA chain propagation. Virology, *63:* 168-175.

Watson, J. D. 1972. Origin of concatemeric T7 DNA. Nature New Biol., *239:* 197-201.

Winnacker, E.-L. 1974. Origins and termini of adenovirus type 2 DNA replication. Cold Spring Harbor Symp. Quant. Biol., *39:* 547-550.

Winnacker, E.-L. 1975. Adenovirus type 2 DNA replication. I. Evidence for discontinuous DNA synthesis. J. Virol., *15:* 744-758.

Wolfson, J., and D. Dressler. 1972. Adenovirus-2 DNA contains an inverted terminal repetition. Proc. Nat. Acad. Sci. U.S., *69:* 3054-3057.

Yamashita, T., and M. Green. 1974. Adenovirus DNA replication. I. Requirement for protein synthesis and isolation of nuclear membrane fractions containing newly synthesized viral DNA and proteins. J. Virol., *14:* 412-420.

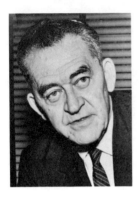

Dr. J. W. Beard
Colloquium Leader

Joseph Beard has been a leader in tumor virus research dating back to 1932 when he started his studies on the rabbit papilloma virus. He has received many honors for his leadership in cancer research. At Duke University he was honored as a James B. Duke Professor of Surgery, and most recently he was given the first award of the Special Virus Cancer Program of the National Cancer Institute in recognition of his outstanding research and his role in the development of the field of virus-related cancer.

Dr. Beard organized at Duke University one of the first meetings of investigators studying virus-induced cancer. This was a small group of about 15 people from various institutes in the United States. Today it is impossible to determine the number of people working in this research area, but it can be said that many of the concepts and means of current investigation have their origin in those early times in the laboratory of Dr. Beard. His devotion to research and determination to discover the role of virus in tumor formation can be demonstrated by his more than 300 publications; and perhaps more significant is his most recent contribution, at the age of 73, which was published this year in *Cancer Research*. This man has not allowed time to leave him behind.

In this short space the editors have not attempted to list Dr. Beard's accomplishments and awards over the past 50 years. We would like only to point out his pioneer role in medical research and his remarkable achievement of being able to stand today as an active contributor to science, a profession where many investigators become victims of the progress they create. Cancer research owes much to this man.

The Editors

Appendix

Thirty-fourth Annual Biology Colloquium

Theme: The Biology of Tumor Viruses

Dates: April 26-27, 1973

Place: Oregon State University, Corvallis, Oregon

Colloquium Committee: George S. Beaudreau, chairman; Richard H. Converse, John A. Kiger, D. D. Kliewer, Roy O. Morris, George D. Pearson, Joe C. Reinert, Stanley P. Snyder

Standing Committee for the Biology Colloquium: J. Ralph Shay, chairman; Robert R. Becker, John R. Dilworth, Robert F. Doerge, Ernst J. Dornfeld, Paul R. Elliker, Betty E. Hawthorne, Charles B. Miller, Knud G. Swenson, John A. Wiens, David L. Willis

Colloquium Speakers, 1973

Joseph W. Beard, Duke University Medical Center, Durham, North Carolina, leader

Dani P. Bolognesi, Duke University Medical Center, Durham, North Carolina

Robert R. Friis, University of Southern California Medical School, Los Angeles, California

Jonathan P. Leis, Duke University Medical Center, Durham, North Carolina

John E. Newbold, University of North Carolina, Durham, North Carolina

George D. Pearson, Oregon State University, Corvallis, Oregon

Special Manuscript Editor: Anne O. Deeney

Cover Illustration: Electron micrography by Ursula Heine of the National Cancer Institute

Sponsorship:

Oregon Division, American Cancer Society

Corvallis Clinic Foundation

Oregon State University

Sigma Xi	Environmental Health Sciences Center
Phi Kappa Phi	Department of Veterinary Medicine
School of Science	Convocations and Lectures Committee
School of Agriculture	Research Council

229   6 1677